EYES ONLY

EYES ONLY

Kenneth B. Kauvar, M.D.
Denver, Colorado

ACC

APPLETON-CENTURY-CROFTS/Norwalk, Connecticut

The author and publisher of this book have taken care to make certain that recommendations regarding treatment and use of drugs are correct and compatible with the standards generally accepted at the time of publication. However, as new information becomes available, changes in treatment and in the use of drugs may become necessary. The reader is urged to consult his or her physician for professional advice in dealing with any serious or potentially serious ophthalmologic problem.

83 84 85 86 / 10 9 8 7 6 5 4 3 2

Prentice-Hall International, Inc., London
Prentice-Hall of Australia, Pty. Ltd., Sydney
Prentice-Hall of India Private Limited, New Delhi
Prentice-Hall of Japan, Inc., Tokyo
Prentice-Hall of Southeast Asia (Pte.) Ltd., Singapore
Whitehall Books Ltd., Wellington, New Zealand

Library of Congress Cataloging in Publication Data

Kauvar, Kenneth B., 1947–
Eyes only.
Includes index.
1. Eye—Diseases and defects. I. Title.
RE48.K34 617.7 82-1833
ISBN 0-8385-2498-2 AACR2

Cover and Text design: Jean M. Sabato

PRINTED IN THE UNITED STATES OF AMERICA

For my family

Contents

Preface

The idea for this book developed over a period of several years from discussions with my patients. Since then I have used brief written descriptions of various common eye problems to supplement and clarify the information I give my patients orally. This book is an expansion of these discussions and descriptions. Since many patients often have the same questions, this book represents my attempt to place the answers to these more frequently asked questions in one comprehensive, convenient format.

Most of the more common eye problems are discussed; however, this book is not intended to cover every condition nor every aspect of any given eye problem. It is not a manual for self-diagnosis and treatment. Rather, the aim is to give an overview of the care of our eyes and the conditions that can adversely affect the well-being of this vital part of the human body.

Since many problems in ophthalmology do not at first appear to be serious, but can, in fact, actually be quite severe, it is important to seek competent help in the event of any persistent problem. New ideas, techniques, and treatments may be introduced in the field that will affect some of the statements in ophthalmology, however, your own ophthalmologist remains a good source of current information and you should not hesitate to ask him or her any questions you may have.

It is my belief that a patient has a right and even an obligation to understand problems that affect him or her to the extent that he or she is interested and able. I hope that this book is one step toward this end in the area of eye care.

Acknowledgments

I would like to thank my patients for asking the questions that have formed the basis of this book, and my teachers for helping me learn the answers. I would also like to thank my agent, Elise Goodman, of Goodman Associates, who thought the idea was worth pursuing; my editor, Doreen Berne, of Appleton-Century-Crofts, who helped make the book more readable; and my secretaries, Donnarae Cody, who would really rather have been doing calligraphy, and Ellen Struthers, who would really rather have been dancing ballet.

CHAPTER 1

Caring for Your Eyes

ANATOMY OF THE EYE

The eye is an organ that focuses incoming light waves onto sensitive nerves. These nerves transmit this information to certain parts of the brain, which in turn interpret them to give the sensation of sight. To say that the act of "seeing" is a complex and amazing process is an understatement.

Basically, light waves coming into the eye must be bent (the technical term is *refracted*) in such a way that they come to a point that focuses on the nerves at the back of the eye. There are two main tissues that bend the incoming light, called the *cornea* and the *lens* (see Fig. 1). These are both living tissues composed of many types of cells, as are the other parts of the eye; all of these tissues need different and specific types of nourishment to function optimally.

Depending on the length of the eye, the cornea and lens may need to supply different amounts of focusing power. The total amount of power needed for the eye to focus light may be provided in different ratios. If the power of the cornea and the lens is not exactly correlated to the length of the eye, one is said to have a

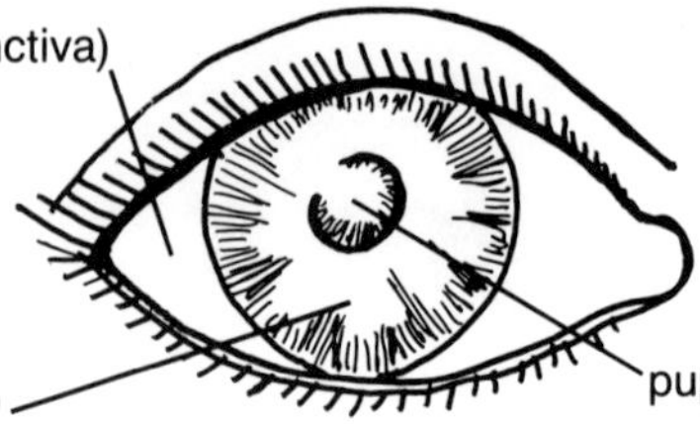

FIGURE 1. Frontal view of the eye. One can see the cornea, iris, and pupil. The lens is behind the iris.

refractive error and glasses are prescribed to compensate for this difference. (Refractive errors are discussed in detail in Chapter 2.)

The cornea is the clear front surface of the eye, and its power is primarily determined by its shape. This shape normally does not change very much. It lies over the pigmented part of the eye which is called the *iris*. Behind the iris is the lens. The lens is suspended in position by thin strands of tissue called *zonules*. The *ciliary muscle* acts on the zonules to change the shape and thus the power of the lens, which is about the size of an aspirin tablet (see Fig. 2). The space behind the lens is filled with a clear jelly-like fluid called *vitreous humor*. (The vitreous humor is discussed further in Chapter 5.)

Between the lens and the cornea, that is, in front of the lens, there is a solution called the *aqueous humor*. The aqueous humor bathes the front part of the lens, the iris, and the back part of the cornea. The space between the iris and the cornea is called the *anterior chamber*. (See Chapter 4 and the discussion of glaucoma.)

In the center of the iris is a circular opening called the *pupil*. Pupil size is enlarged by the *dilator muscle* and decreased by the *constrictor muscle*. The size of the pupil opening is important in a number of ways. In bright light, the pupil constricts to allow *less* light in, and in the dark it dilates to allow *more* light in. When the pupil is dilated (as at night) light waves that normally would not have been

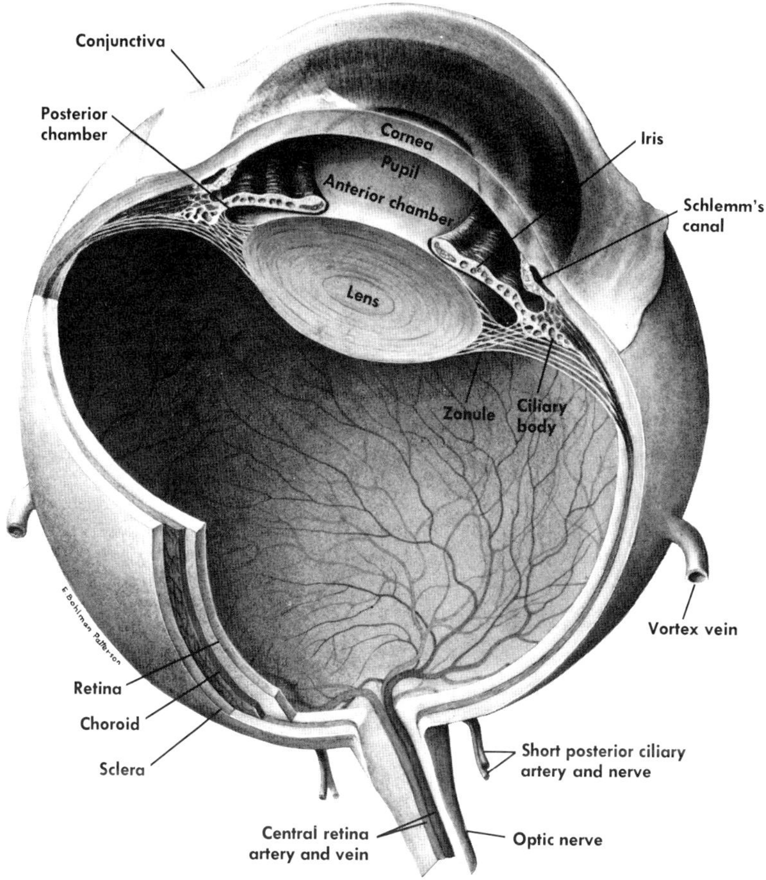

FIGURE 2. Cross-section of the eye. This is a diagram of an eye with the outer part removed. The various parts are labelled. In addition, one can see the relative size and location of the lens, vitreous cavity, retina, and optic nerve. (Modified from Frank W. Newell and Terry Ernest, *Ophthalmology: Principles and Concepts,* 3rd ed. Copyright 1974, C. V. Mosby Co., St. Louis, p. 34)

able to pass through the lens are now allowed to pass through. This leads to a slight change in refraction, which in most people is not noticeable. In those individuals for whom this difference is apparent, the phenomenon is called night myopia and sometimes can be corrected with a different eyeglass prescription. In some people, opacities in the lens that were covered by the iris are exposed to incoming light waves when the pupil is dilated. This can cause a dazzle effect, particularly when looking directly at a light, such as oncoming car headlights. The light bounces off the opacities in different directions and creates the dazzle. (See Chapter 4 and the discussion of *cataracts.*)

The nerves on which the light is focused are contained in a tissue called the *retina.* These nerves are connected directly to the brain. The retina, with the nerves, lines the back of the eye. It is a thin tissue, about the same thickness as a facial tissue. (See Chapters 4 and 5 for further discussion of the retina and specific eye problems.)

All of the extensions of the nerves of the retina leave the eye in one large bundle of approximately 1 million smaller nerves called the *optic nerve.* The optic nerve connects with other nerves of the brain.

The eyeball itself is roughly a sphere about one inch in diameter. There are six muscles on the outside of the eye that move the eye from side to side and up and down. The eye can also rotate slightly. These muscles normally keep both eyes properly aligned (see Fig. 3). When they are misaligned, certain problems develop. (See the section on *strabismus* in Chapter 3.)

The eye is surrounded by bones with a cushion of fat between the bones and the eye, except in the front where the lids protect the eye by covering it.

These various tissues and their functions are discussed in more detail in the rest of the book, along with various emergency and preventive measures.

THE EYE EXAMINATION

A general eye examination by an ophthalmologist can include a number of different steps. A history is obtained first. Identifying information, your occupation, and major complaint are noted. Your

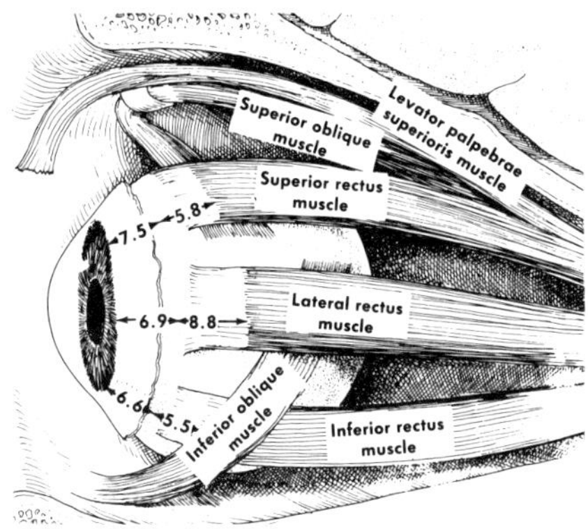

FIGURE 3. Extraocular muscles. This view shows the eye from the side. Five of the six muscles that are on the outside of the eye are shown. The medial rectus muscle is in the same position as the lateral rectus muscle, except on the other side of the eye. One of the muscles to the upper eyelid is also shown. (From Frank W. Newell and Terry Ernest, *Ophthalmology: Principles and Concepts,* 3rd ed. Copyright 1974, C. V. Mosby Co., St. Louis, p. 34.)

occupation may be important for a number of reasons. For example, a musician may need to read clearly at a different distance than a draftsman. Any previous problems including any injuries, infections, or surgery on your eyes are also noted. Medications that you take, allergies to drugs, and any other medical problems you have should be mentioned to the physician. If anyone in your family has had an eye problem it should be discussed. For each symptom you have, it is important to describe it and to tell when it started, how fast it changed, and if anything made it better or worse.

Determining Visual Acuity

The actual examination requires your cooperation and participation for the most accurate results. There is generally no pain or real discomfort in an eye examination. How well you see, or *visual acuity,* is determined for each eye by reading a standard eye chart, composed of letters of the alphabet. For people who are not familiar with the English alphabet, or small children, other charts are available with the letter E pointing in different directions or with pictures of common objects (see Fig. 4). Acuity is recorded by a shorthand notation, with normal recorded as 20/20. Acuity of 20/40 is still quite good. It does *not* mean that your vision is half as good as someone with 20/20 vision. The first number gives the distance the patient is from the chart and the second number gives the distance at which a

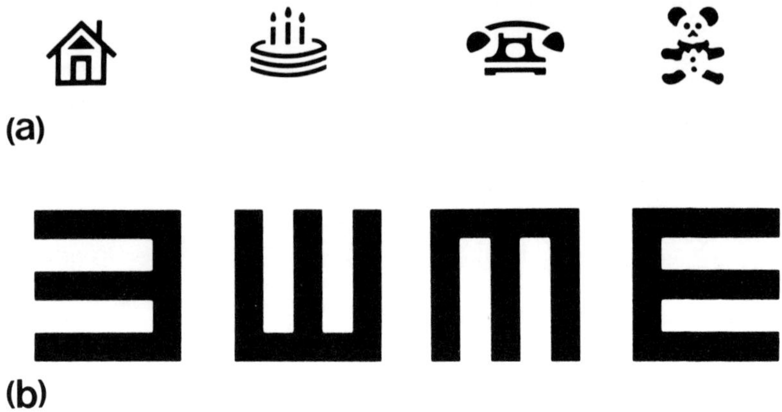

FIGURE 4. Charts for testing vision in children. Picture cards (Henry F. Allen preschool vision test) of this sort (a) or an E facing in different directions (b) can be used to test the visual acuity of young children or people who speak only a foreign language. The size of the objects can be varied just as the more commonly used alphabet letters.

patient with normal vision would still be able to see the letter. For example, 20/30 vision means that the patient is 20 feet from the chart and that a person with normal vision could see the same letter from a distance of 30 feet. (Six meters is about the same as 20 feet and for people using the metric system 6/6 would be normal vision. Some doctors do not have an office 20 feet long and in those cases a system of mirrors is used to obtain the necessary distance.) The patient with 20/30 vision, however, must be 20 feet from the chart to see a letter on the 20/30 line. Visual acuity better than normal could be recorded as 20/15. This would mean that the letter could be seen from 20 feet, while a normal person would need to be 15 feet away to distinguish it. Such acuity is sometimes seen in younger individuals.

This number only measures your visual acuity. There are other important aspects of your eyesight that it does not refer to, such as the visual field. Your best corrected vision is what counts, that is, your vision with proper eyeglasses is the important measurement.

Refraction Examination

In order to determine the proper power eyeglasses, a refraction examination is performed. This determination, depending on your visual acuity and eyeglasses prescription, may involve both objective and subjective measurements. Objective measurements are determined by shining a light in your eye and noting how it is reflected with different lenses placed in front of your eye, a technique called *retinoscopy*. Subjective measurements are made by giving you two sets of lenses to look through and asking you which set is better. A different set of lenses is used each time, although many will look similar (see Fig. 5). Two choices are always given and they are designated in a given way. There is no right or wrong answer. In fact, sometimes both choices may be somewhat blurred. You just need to pick the lens that is clearer to you, or say if they are about the same.

It is important to determine your refractive error when you are looking at far-off distances, that is, when the mechanism that allows you to focus closer is completely relaxed. For this reason, a distance of 20 feet is chosen and special eye drops are frequently used to prevent you from focusing on closer objects. The time of maximum effect of the eye drops depends on many factors such as the type of drop chosen and the individual person's response. Younger patients need different drops. These may take longer to soak in and may last somewhat longer. With the drops, you should still be able to see far away and to drive home if you were able to drive *to* the office. Sunglasses may be needed if it is bright outside, since the drops also keep your pupils dilated. Disposable sunglasses are generally available on request if you did not bring your own. The time that it takes for the drops to wear off depends on the type of drop, the amount used, and the individual person, but generally they start to wear off within 24 hours. Drops to reverse the first effect are generally not used since the individual then has to contend with the second drop's actions, side effects, time of onset, and time of elimination as well.

In addition to measurement of your refractive error, observation is made of the side-to-side and up-and-down motions of your eyes to see if they move in a normal range and if they work together properly. A shield may be placed alternately over one eye to see if

FIGURE 5. Phoropter. A phoropter is an instrument that has various lenses built into it and, by rotating different dials, different lenses can be brought into the patient's line of sight.

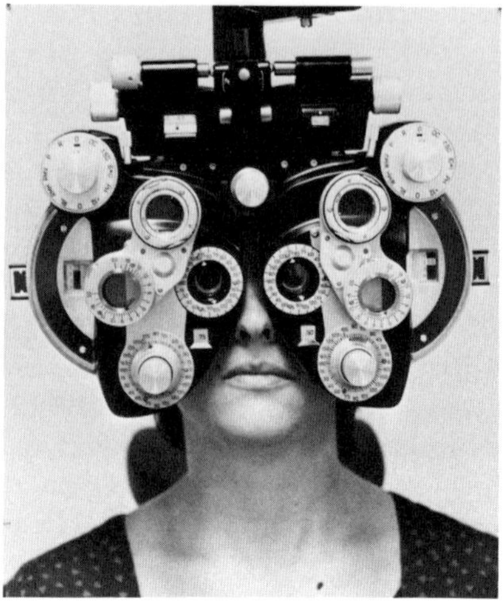

there is any drift. The reaction of your pupils to a single light is also noted, and the quality of your visual field may be observed in a number of ways. (Visual field is discussed in Chapter 4 in the section on glaucoma.)

Eye Pressure and Glaucoma Examination

A special microscope with an adjustable light beam is used to examine various parts of your eye. This instrument is called a *slit lamp* (see Fig. 6). It is utilized with another instrument in checking internal eye pressure which may be high if you have glaucoma.

In order to get the various parts of your eye in focus, the instrument is movable to a certain degree. The width, angle, intensity, and color of the beam can be varied, allowing the observer to see different locations more easily. A local anesthetic eye drop, a topical dye, and a blue light are generally used to allow better visualization of the pressure scale. It is important that you cooperate by keeping your chin in the chin rest with your forehead firmly against the head rest so that your head remains perfectly still and your eyes do not drift out of focus. (See Figs. 7, 8) When using this microscope to measure the pressure inside your eyes, the ophthalmologist is also determining

FIGURE 6. Slit lamp. This instrument has a number of features. There are observer eyepieces that produce magnification. A light whose direction, width, length, intensity, and color can be varied is used to obtain different views of the eye. The instrument can also be positioned at different heights and distances from various parts of the eye in order to focus on different areas.

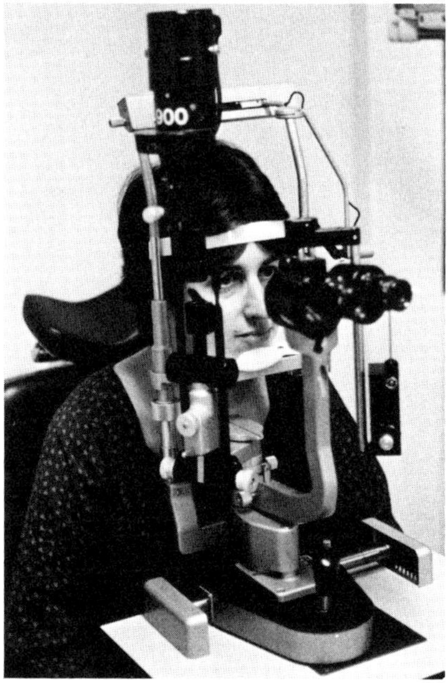

whether or not you may be developing glaucoma. Measuring internal eye pressure is a common technique for checking for glaucoma.

You should not rub your eyes too vigorously after this part of the examination because it takes about 30 minutes to one hour for the local anesthetic to wear off and you could rub too hard, not feel it, and cause injury.

Other instruments used for measuring eye pressure are the Schiotz tonometer, an electronic tonometer, and a tonometer that uses a puff of air. The former does not require an anesthetic drop and can be used by non-physicians as a screening technique.

Ophthalmoscopy

In order to look completely at the nerves and blood vessels lining the back of your eye (called the *fundus*), it is generally necessary to use eye drops to dilate your pupils. Many of the most effective dilating drops also cause you to have some difficulty focusing on objects

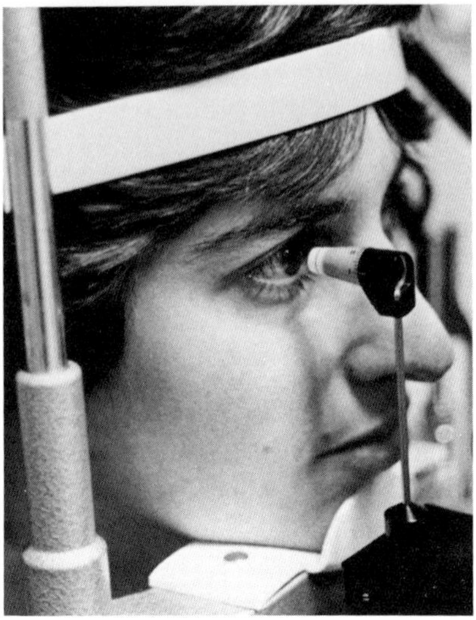

FIGURE 7. Applanation tonometer. This instrument, in conjunction with the slit lamp, is used to measure the pressure inside the eye, called the *intraocular pressure.* This is not the same as blood pressure.

closer than a few feet away, as previously discussed. This examination technique is called *ophthalmoscopy,* and an ophthalmoscope is used to perform it.

Other Eye Tests

A variety of other procedures and examination techniques are available, if indicated, for specific purposes, such as measuring the curvature of your cornea for help in determining refractive error or for contact lens fitting. A special contact lens, called a three-mirror lens, used with a local anesthetic and the slit lamp, may be used to get a different view of the nerves and blood vessels or other parts of your eye. Color vision, stereoscopic vision, and fusion ability may also be tested.

Preventive Aspects of the Eye Exam

A complete medical eye examination, as described previously, may also detect signs of other diseases. For example, diseases that affect blood vessels such as hypertension or diabetes may have manifestations in the blood vessels of the back of the eye. A problem with the brain, such as an abnormality of a blood vessel or a tumor, may

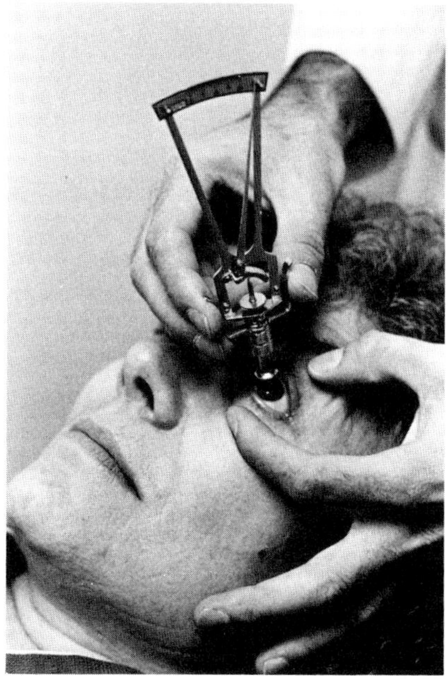

FIGURE 8. Schiotz tonometer. This is another instrument for measuring intraocular pressure.

produce changes in the appearance of the nerves, eye movements, or pupil reactions before other signs of a problem become apparent. In addition, many problems that affect other parts of the body also affect the eyes. Examples include collagen diseases, sarcoidosis, and pituitary problems. It is important for the examiner to understand these other problems in order to properly care for the eye. In medical school and subsequent training, an ophthalmologist learns about these and many other medical problems that affect other parts of the body as well as the eyes.

An internist or family physician can also detect some problems in the eye itself or some ocular manifestations of general disease.

Frequency of Checkups

How often a general examination is needed depends on many factors, including such things as your age, current problem, and family history. Each case is different, but generally an eye exam every one to two years is sufficient if you have no particular problem or complaint. Some doctors, if you prefer, will send postcards to remind you of the time for your next appointment. Signs of possible eye trouble in children that should signal a visit to the eye doctor include such things as rubbing the eyes excessively, visual complaints, squinting, crossed eyes, or infections. Children should have at least a vision test every year. These are usually given in school screening programs. Other screening programs, such as those for measuring internal eye pressure, are sponsored from time to time by various groups at health fairs and other community events. While these screening examinations do accomplish some aspects of a general eye examination, one should not assume that normal results of one or a few isolated tests mean that there are no other problems with your eyes. Even an abnormal result may not be significant. An eye examination should be scheduled if there is any question about either an adult or child, since some problems cannot be treated as effectively if they are discovered later. It is also possible to examine very young children, even infants, if there is any question about the well-being of the child's eyes.

An eye examination can be fun for children, and not associated with fear, as the following case illustrates:

Case 1

Sally was a young girl who was coming for her first eye examination. She didn't like going to doctors because there was generally pain associated with it. Recent experiences included immunization shots at the pediatrician's office and a cavity filling at the dentist's office. Now she was coming to the ophthalmologist's office. Fortunately, her mother had tried to prepare her for the experience. She emphasized the positive aspects, telling Sally that it would be fun and there would be games to play with the doctor. She did not mention anything about pain. She never said "It won't hurt." Sally practiced pointing her fingers in the same direction as the fingers of the E that her mother held in different orientations. Her mother gave her a lot of positive reinforcement by telling her how well she was doing with this game. She never mentioned anything about getting one wrong. If she did get one wrong, her mother simply said she was doing well and asked if another direction was better. Sally would agree and move her fingers accordingly.

When Sally came in for the examination she was excited. She looked forward to playing the game she had learned at home. She was interested in all the gadgets and lights. When it came time for the eye drops she was told that some people ask for a few extra ones because they like them so much. After she had the drops inserted, she decided she was not one of those people. She was directed to the waiting room and was distracted from the eye drop experience by the games in the waiting room. After the drops soaked in, she came back "to play more games." She left the office smiling and proudly wearing her very own pair of disposable sunglasses.

EYE CARE PROVIDERS

Ophthalmologists

The eye examination just described is generally what an ophthalmologist will do. The examinations by an optician or optometrist are not as comprehensive, as they are trained differently.

It is important to understand who an *ophthalmologist* is. After graduating from high school, an ophthalmologist attends college, generally spending four years there and obtaining a bachelor of arts (B.A.) or bachelor of science (B.S.) degree. After college, he or she attends medical school, which takes an additional four or sometimes five years, to obtain a doctor of medicine (M.D.) degree. Generally, after graduation from medical school the ophthalmologist spends one year as an intern where he or she takes care of hospitalized patients, covers the emergency room, and has a clinic. This is followed by three or more years of ophthalmology residency, during which the doctor concentrates specifically on problems of the eye, in addition to learning surgical techniques. After that, one or more years of additional fellowship training may be taken to concentrate study on a specific part of the eye, such as the cornea or the retina. Thus, an ophthalmologist spends considerable time learning about other parts of the body, as well as about many diseases and drugs not now thought to affect the eye directly (but which may be found to do so in the future), in addition to studying those diseases and drugs that are known to directly affect the eye.

An ophthalmologist is a physician who specializes in the total care of the eyes and is referred to as a doctor. Ophthalmologists are trained to give a comprehensive medical eye examination in order to diagnose disorders and diseases of the eye and to carry out the medical and surgical procedures necessary for their treatment. This would include examining for refractive errors; prescribing and fitting eyeglasses, low-vision aids, and contact lenses; prescribing exercises and orthoptic training; using both topical and systemic drugs; and treating injuries, in addition to performing surgical procedures when indicated.

Optometrists and Opticians

There is another profession concerned with examination of the eyes, *optometry*. After graduating from high school an optometrist spends from two to four years in college, followed by four years in optometry school to obtain a doctor of optometry (O.D.) degree. An optometrist is trained to examine eyes to detect refractive errors and some other diseases; to prescribe glasses, low-vision aids, and contact lenses; and to prescribe exercises. In some states optometrists may use certain topical drugs. If an optometrist has a patient with another type of eye problem or one who needs surgery, he will refer the patient to an ophthalmologist. An optometrist is also referred to as a doctor even though the training is different.

An *optician* is trained to fill the prescriptions for eyeglasses that either an ophthalmologist or an optometrist prescribes. An optician takes care that appropriate frames are chosen and that the lenses are ground correctly and fit into the frames properly. The optician also adjusts the frames to fit on the face. He or she can repair damaged frames and may have low-vision aids available.

The Well-Prepared Patient

Keep a list of any questions you have so that you can remember to ask them when you speak with your ophthalmologist. Never be afraid to ask any question, as silly as you may think it is. It is important that you understand your particular problem, so please ask if there is something you don't understand or wonder about.

MEDICATIONS

What to Tell the Doctor

As a general rule, it is most helpful, and frequently quite necessary, for any doctor you visit to know exactly what medicines you have been taking. This includes medicines that may not seem to be directly related to the problem for which you came to that particular doctor. Medicines applied to one part of the body or taken orally can sometimes affect your eyes, since they are absorbed into your bloodstream and distributed throughout your system. For example, an undesired side effect of high doses of prednisone over long periods of time can be cataract formation, and of chloroquine, retinal problems. Some drugs used to treat intestinal spasm can cause acute glaucoma in certain susceptible individuals.

Similarly, eye drops can affect other parts of your body. For example, timolol, which is one of the drugs used to treat glaucoma, can cause respiratory problems in certain individuals. Furthermore, sometimes one drug can interact with another drug to cause a problem, so-called drug-drug interactions. Any previous allergic reaction to any medicines should also be noted, along with what the reaction was. If there is any question about the name of the drug you are taking, bring the bottle with the medicine in it. It is also helpful for you to bring in your old eyeglasses, even if they are broken, or your old prescription, if you have it.

Drop and Ointment Insertion

Eye drops and ointments are specially formulated for your eyes. The same drug in, for example, an antibiotic ointment preparation for your skin, should *not* be used for your eyes since the vehicle the drug is dissolved in is different and may be harmful to them.

Before inserting eye drops you should wash your hands thoroughly. Carefully remove the top and place it on a clean tissue. Keep the tip of the bottle from touching your fingers, lashes, or anything else.

The easiest way to insert eye drops is to pull the lower lid down and out a little bit, pulling the skin *gently* with the forefinger of one hand. Hold the bottle between the thumb and forefinger of the other hand, bracing the other fingers against the side of your nose. Tilt your head back, look up, and put one drop in the pouch between the lid and the eyeball. Then gently close and blink. An ointment should be inserted similarly, except instead of a drop, place a ribbon of ointment in the lower pouch, look down, and then gently close the eyes. Wash your hands after applying the medication (see Fig. 9).

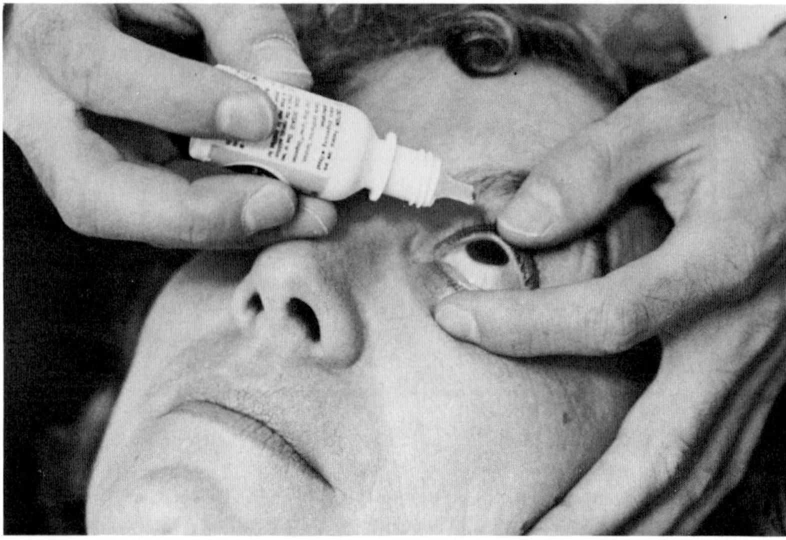

FIGURE 9. Eye drop and ointment application. The easiest way to apply an eye drop is to pull down gently on the lower lid, look up, and place the drop in the small sac-like area (called the cul-de-sac) between the lower lid and the eyeball. Then gently close the lid. This method usually prevents the blink reflex from blocking the drop and is also more comfortable since the drop is not being dropped directly on the cornea; which is more sensitive. An ointment is applied the same way. A single ribbon of ointment placed across the cul-de-sac is usually sufficient. If both a drop and ointment are to be applied, use the drop first, wait a few minutes, and then place the ointment in. If two or more drops are to be used, it is best to wait a few minutes between the drops to prevent overflow onto the cheek.

If a patch needs to be removed it should be done by first pulling the tape from the forehead and then removing the part over the cheek.

One should be careful when inserting medications in the eye. If the eye is infected, for example, one can spread the infection to the other eye by touching the infected eye and then rubbing the normal one. Another type of problem is illustrated by the following case:

Case 2

Catherine A. was a woman about 30 years old who had an inflammation in one eye. Part of her treatment included the use of long-acting dilating drops for that eye. The other eye was normal. After she had been on treatment for a week or so, she came in complaining of blurred vision in the previously normal eye. She was afraid, and so was I, that the inflammation had spread.

Examination revealed no inflammation in the second eye, but this eye was also widely dilated. I decided that she probably transferred some of the eye drop solution to this eye by getting it on her fingers or using a facial tissue. I reassured her and some days later the medication wore off and the second eye was back to normal.

COMMON MISCONCEPTIONS ABOUT EYE CARE

There are many ideas that people commonly share about their eyes; however, many of them are no longer considered true. Although some of them were thought correct at one time, proper experiments and research have proven otherwise. Of course, it is possible that at some future point, with new knowledge, different ideas will replace current ones as true. Until then, however, one must accept what is presently known and proven in a given field as correct, and use that as the basis for appropriate behavior.

Each of the ideas in the following list is discussed in a later section or chapter. You can test your understanding of these ideas in advance, by deciding whether each statement is true or false.

1. You can severely damage your eyes by using a light that is too dim.
2. You can severely damage your eyes by sitting too close to a television set or by holding a book too close to your eyes.
3. A contact lens in ordinary use can get lost behind the eye.
4. If you wear contact lenses for a prescribed period of time, you will no longer need to wear contact lenses or glasses because you will have eliminated your refractive error.

5. If you need glasses to see clearly things that are far away, you will outgrow this problem.
6. It is important to change your glasses every year, even if there is only a small change in the prescription.
7. If a middle-aged person who needs glasses to see far away can read better by taking his glasses off, his eyes are better than another middle-aged person who needs reading glasses or bifocals to read.
8. A cataract is a film that is peeled off during surgery.
9. The time to operate on a cataract is the same for every person.
10. Your eyes will "wear out" if you use them too much, or if you only have one, it will wear out faster.
11. If you need glasses to see clearly, you can eliminate this need by resting your eyes periodically and doing exercises.
12. It is important for everyone to use an eyewash every day.
13. Headaches are almost always caused by a problem with the eyes.
14. If your eyes are definitely crossed, you can usually outgrow the problem.
15. Makeup never causes problems with one's eyes.
16. During a cataract operation, the eyeball is removed from the head and later placed back in position.
17. During an eye operation, the eye being operated on can "see" what is being done.
18. When local anesthesia is used, the initial injections are given directly into the eye.
19. For a corneal transplant to be successful it is necessary to use a donor cornea from a person of the same age, sex, and eye color.
20. Glaucoma goes away if you ignore it, especially if you don't notice any pain and think you see normally.
21. Eye exercises generally help resolve reading problems.
22. Cataracts are caused by using your eyes too much.
23. Most people with glaucoma go blind, even when treated appropriately.
24. Incorrect glasses for an adult cause irreversible damage to the eyes as opposed to being simply uncomfortable.

25. It is never necessary to rest your eyes, even after reading for a long period of time at one sitting.*

EMERGENCY PROCEDURES

It is important to know what to do in an emergency situation without having to ask someone or refer to a book. Frequently there is not enough time to call for help because some steps should be taken immediately.

One of the most commonly occurring emergencies is when foreign material accidentally enters the eye. This is discussed in the following sections in terms of the kind of material or object and the appropriate treatment for each.

Powders and Chemicals

In cases where laundry soap powder or liquid, chalk from marking lines on a playing field, chemical solutions, or solid particles of chemicals such as bathroom drain cleaner have entered the eye(s), the most important thing is to rinse the eye out immediately with the nearest source of water as continuously as possible for at least 15 minutes. Swiftness of treatment is the critical factor. *Every second counts.* The lids must be open and the eyeball itself must be in contact with the water. Do *not* try to prepare or use special solutions since they can be more harmful than good. Use plain water, and a lot of it. You can put your head (or the affected person's) under a faucet with lukewarm (if you have a choice) water or even a garden hose, or you can fill a glass with water and pour it on the eye. Then call an ophthalmologist, or have someone else call one while you are rinsing the eye. *Rinse first and then call.*

If it is difficult to keep the lids open and professional help can be obtained within 15 minutes, irrigate for five minutes and go immediately to the nearest emergency room or ophthalmologist's

**Answers:* Every one of the listed statements is false, that is, none of them is true. If you have a question about any one of them, please continue reading. If, after finishing this book, you still have a question, ask your ophthalmologist, who should be able to give a more extensive explanation.

office, where additional techniques can be used to ensure adequate irrigation. The following case illustrates how this knowledge should be used:

Case 3

Jimmy W. was playing soccer in school one afternoon when he fell near the boundary line. As he looked up, other people were also falling and dust mixed with chalk from the boundary marking line was kicked into his face and eyes. He felt intense stinging in his eyes. Luckily for Jimmy, the people with him realized what had happened and knew they should immediately begin washing out his eyes. The bucket of drinking water with paper cups was used. His mother brought him to me for treatment shortly after the incident. He had had about five minutes of irrigation to his eyes, but was having difficulty keeping them open.

I used anesthetic drops and continued to flush out Jimmy's eyes for another 10 minutes. I everted his lids and removed chalk particles that were embedded there. I then treated his corneal abrasions and placed eye patches. The next day when the patches were removed Jimmy felt fine and had nearly normal vision. His vision was completely normal a few days later. He was grateful that his friends knew what to do immediately after the injury as he has since heard of people who were not so fortunate.

Metals and Other Solid Objects

Other types of material that may enter the eye cannot be rinsed out as one can rinse a powder or a liquid. Examples include a piece of metal chipped from an axe or from grinding or filing, or shattered glass fragments. In these cases it is important to leave the eye alone and to call an ophthalmologist for immediate treatment. Unless chemical solutions have also gotten into the eye, do not try to rinse or rub the material out, since you may spread the material around and push it further into the eye. If, however, chemical solutions have also entered the eye, you should rinse with water as described in the previous section. Special care should be taken to avoid pushing on the eyeball itself. This is particularly important when opening the lid. It is possible to open the lid and push it against the surrounding bone to keep the eye open, thus avoiding pressure on the eyeball.

Sometimes a dust particle or an eyelash gets under the upper eyelid. It is fairly easy to lift up the upper lid. This is done by pulling the lid away from the globe by gently pulling on the lashes, then pushing in with a finger or cotton-tipped applicator above the lash margin while the other hand flips the lid over (see Fig. 10). Often the particle can be flicked out with a piece of tissue or by irrigating with water. However, this eversion of the lid should *never* be attempted if there is any question that the eyeball itself has been cut or penetrated.

Blows to the Orbit

If you are hit around the eye, for example, by a racquet or a fist, you should immediately apply cold compresses to the area for 15 minutes and then every hour or so for the first day, except when sleeping. Since much of the swelling is caused by leaking from damaged blood vessels, reducing the blood flow by the use of cold compresses also reduces the swelling. Since the area around the eye is limited by the bones of the orbit, there is not much room for swelling. Thus, excessive swelling can be painful and cause damaging pressure on the nerves of the eye. However, excessive treatment with cold can also cause damage by reducing blood flow too much. An ophthalmologist should be called to arrange an examination to determine if there has been damage to the inside of your eye.

Even seemingly trivial injuries can be accompanied by a small perforation of the eyeball or penetration of a small foreign body to the inside of the eyeball. There may be a small amount of bleeding that is easy for an untrained observer to overlook. Residual particles may be trapped under a lid. These complications can be potentially serious, enough so as to result in complete loss of vision. An ophthalmological examination can generally detect these problems and should not be overlooked.

Cuts Around or Through the Eye

If you are cut in or around the eye, put a light bandage (one that does *not* place pressure on the eye) over the eye and call an ophthalmologist at once. Do *not* try to remove any object that appears to have possibly penetrated into the eye or orbital area. Do *not* manipulate the lids if you suspect the globe may have been perforated.

FIGURE 10. Eyelid eversion technique. Gently pull down and out on the upper eyelashes. Then place a finger or cotton-tipped applicator on the skin (a). Gently push down with the applicator while the other hand pulls the lid out and up (b,c). Note that the eyelid should never be everted if there is any question as to whether the eyeball was cut open or penetrated by an object.

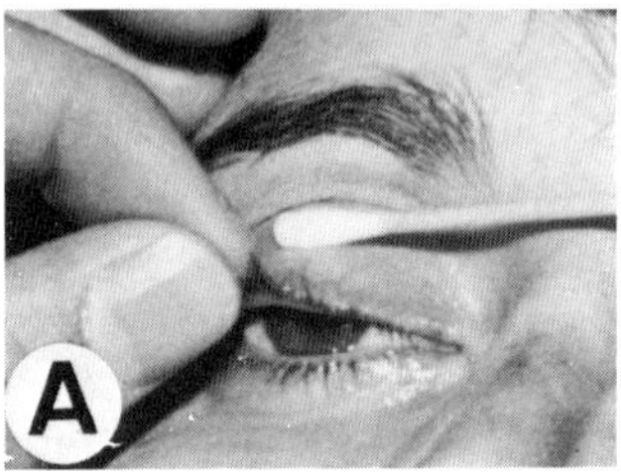

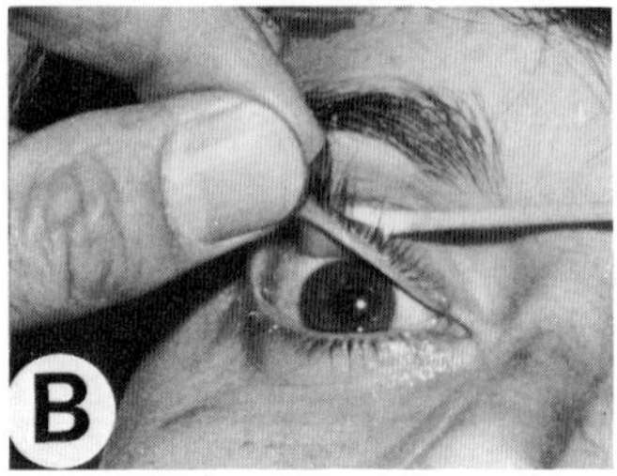

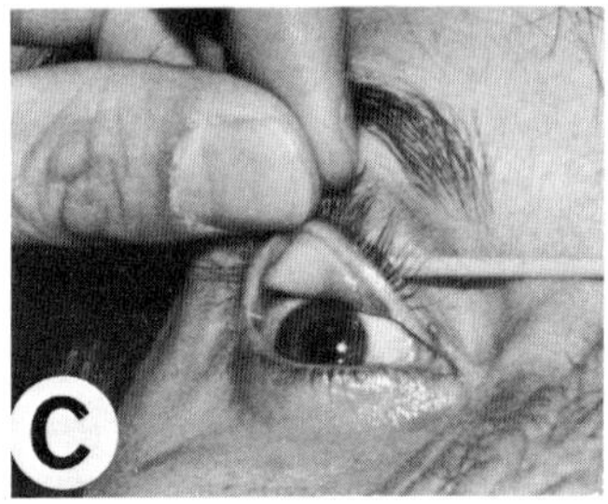

Heat Injuries

Injury from heat requires ophthalmological care. The eye should be gently patched and your physician called immediately.

Changes in Vision

Sudden, persistent changes in vision for no apparent reason and lasting over a few minutes or hours are also emergencies. If you notice a "curtain" coming down or up over your field of vision, you should call an ophthalmologist. Sudden severe pain or discharge also require attention and should not be dismissed by thinking the symptom will go away. It could be serious. A painful red eye with or without loss of vision can be potentially blinding, even though most often it is not serious.

Sudden total loss of vision requires immediate ophthalmological examination. While you are en route to the ophthalmologist's office, breathe into a paper bag or similar container and massage the eye. The reasons for this are discussed in Chapter 6 in the section on central retinal artery occlusion. Sudden persistent drooping of the eyelid should also be evaluated by an ophthalmologist without delay.

Additional Information

It is helpful to have emergency procedure sheets for eye care posted in various locations in the home. Such sticker-sheets as "First Aid for Eye Emergencies" and "How to Jump-Start a Car Safely" are particularly useful. (Battery acid injuries resulting from problems in jump-starting a car are quite common.) These stickers and other useful information are available from the National Society to Prevent Blindness, Inc., 79 Madison Avenue, New York, New York 10016. Telephone: (212) 684-3505. Local chapters exist in many locations.

PREVENTION OF INJURY

Protection from Trauma

About 90 percent of all eye injuries are said to be preventable. Many eye injuries occur from a fall or while participating in various sports. Tennis balls, racquet balls, handballs, and their accompanying racquets can cause severe injury to the eyes, even to the point of blindness. It is imperative that safety goggles or safety glasses with plastic lenses and flexible frames be worn when participating in such activities (see Fig. 11). Polycarbonate and CR-39 are two new types of extremely hard plastic that should be used for safety lenses wherever possible. These plastics are much harder than glass and polycarbonate cannot be shattered even when the lens is placed on the floor and hit directly with a hammer. They are available in most eyeglass prescriptions, and can be made with no power if prescription lenses are not needed. Other conventional plastic lenses designed for safety use may be satisfactory for some purposes, but these two types of plastic are the best where safety and prevention are concerned.

Safety lenses are thicker in the center than regular lenses, so the frames should be appropriate for this use. Frames are available that are more flexible and have hinges that can rotate nearly 360 degrees, along with large rubber nose pieces for added protection. The lenses are placed in the frame in such a way that they will pop out *away* from the eye and not toward it if the impact is sufficiently strong. Eyeguards without a lens are not as safe. A ball traveling at high speed can be compressed enough to penetrate these guards

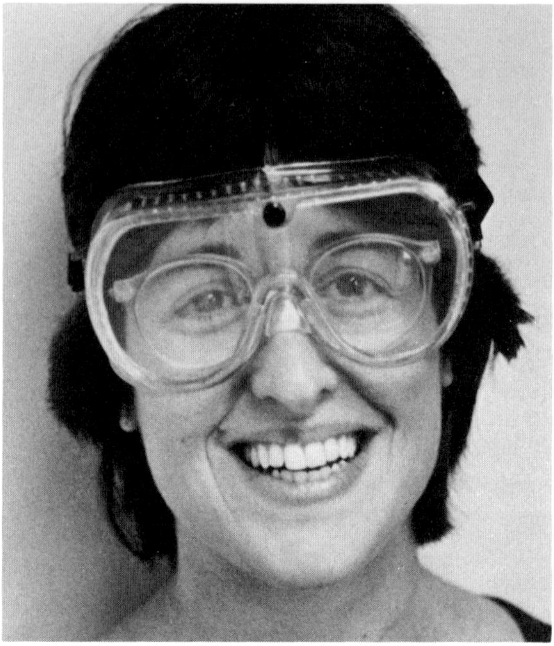

FIGURE 11. Protective gear. A number of different types of protective goggles and glasses are available. It is important is use one appropriate for the work one is doing.

and cause severe damage. In addition, contact lenses are *not* protective and if worn, require additional protection, such as polycarbonate lenses with no power, and frames as already described. Hockey requires a helmet with a face guard that completely protects the eyes. A polyurethane supportive material inside the helmet is better than sponge rubber because it absorbs better and dissipates the force of a blow to the head. A variety of such safety items are available from many opticians. Helmets are available at most sporting goods stores and goggles are available from opticians or hardware stores.

The following case illustrates what can happen when preventive measures are not taken:

Case 4

Robert M. was a star tennis player who played the game quite aggressively. He always rushed the net and was the sort of partner everyone wanted to have when they played doubles. He had excellent vision and did not need to wear glasses to see clearly. Since he did not wear glasses, it did not occur to him to wear eye protection gear. (Sometimes people who wear glasses are more aware of their vulnerability, such as how easily regular frames and lenses can be broken.) One day Robert was playing doubles against an equally aggressive team; his partner was serving. He was at the net and was distracted by a friend arriving to watch the match when he suddenly looked back at the court to see a tennis ball coming straight at his head. He tried to duck but the ball hit him directly in the eye at high speed. He had intense pain.

Robert was taken to see me and I noted some bleeding in his eye with a slightly elevated intraocular pressure. He was told to rest and the eye was observed frequently. The pressure continued to rise and medication was needed to help reduce the pressure. Fortunately for him, the bleeding stopped and the pressure returned to normal. He now wears protective gear when he plays tennis. He also tries not to be distracted when on the court.

In accordance with federal law since 1972, glasses worn for everyday use are treated either by heat or with chemicals to prevent them from shattering into thousands of small fragments. These lenses are termed "impact resistant." However, this does *not* mean that they cannot break. They can still be broken into perhaps three or four larger fragments and the sharp edge can cut an eye. Obviously, regular plastic or metal frames can easily be broken and these fragments can damage the eye. Plastic frames should also be flame resistant. Always inquire at the place where your glasses are made to be certain that the lenses are impact resistant.

Protection from Bright Light

Activities where light intensity is great require adequate sunglasses. Skiing, sailing, or lying on the beach in the bright sun are just a few examples. There is about a four- to eight-hour time lag after excessive sun exposure for the damage and painful symptoms to become noticeable. It should also be noted that it is *never* safe to intentionally look directly at the sun, even during an eclipse, even through sunglasses or exposed film, or with any other technique. Do *not* use lenses to focus the sun indirectly onto paper. Again, the damage is delayed and in this case, is often irreversible.

Sunglasses for general use should transmit no more than 20 to 30 percent of incoming light, that is, they should absorb 70 to 80 percent of incoming light. For such activities as arc welding, glasses or goggles that transmit one percent or less light are needed. Neutral gray, green, or brown are acceptable colors for sunglasses. Sunglasses should *not* be worn when driving at night or when driving in a tunnel.

Some people like phototropic-type lenses that change color depending on the light conditions, but many people find that the five minutes or more that they take to change is inconvenient. In addition, the windshield in a car blocks many of the wavelengths of light that cause the color to change and so they may not be as dark as one would like while driving. This type of lens, even under optimal conditions, will generally not absorb as much light as is desirable, since they are dependent on the surrounding temperature and other factors. They are also more expensive and are not made of plastic. Some people, however, are quite happy with them. Bifocals can be made in this type of lens, if desired.

Clip-on–type sunglasses are acceptable for occasional use, but if sunglasses are worn frequently, optical-quality glass with one's prescription ground into it if one wears corrective eyeglasses is preferable. It is possible to make bifocal sunglasses, if so desired. Some people find polarized sunglasses helpful in reducing glare. A slight tint is also found useful by some people in reducing the glare encountered indoors from fluorescent lights.

Protection in Hazardous Occupations

Activities such as arc welding, machine grinding, or even working under a car should include the use of shields to protect the eyes from stray fragments as part of standard safety precautions, in addition to dark lenses to protect them from high-intensity light, where applicable. If you are working with chemical solutions or aerosols, or even if you are just in an area where they are being used, you also need protective goggles. These safety measures are not just for regular work but also for home repairs and some hobbies. Wearing proper eye protection is not nearly as difficult to get used to as getting used to partial or total blindness! It is not harmful to wear protective lenses or goggles for long periods. Your ophthalmologist can direct you to sources of appropriate protective gear available in your location. You must always insist on being properly protected visually in all situations, as the following case illustrates:

Case 5

George T. was a 34-year-old day laborer who performed many different types of jobs. One day he was assigned to a job that required the use of a power sander. He had had experience with this tool and knew that goggles should be worn when it is used. He asked his employer for goggles and was told that there weren't any and that "they aren't needed." George then noted that a plate that is used to lock the sandpaper in place was missing. He asked his employer about this problem and was told, "It doesn't matter. Use several sheets of sandpaper to fill in the space." George did as he was told and started sanding. Just after he started, the sandpaper tore out of position and he felt something in his eye. He asked his employer where the first aid eyewash was and was told, "There isn't one. Just relax." His employer then left the premises.

George was seen by me in moderate pain. He had sand particles embedded in the center of his cornea. I removed them, but since they were so deep he now has a small scar that distorts his central vision. He has been told that a corneal transplant might help him but he hasn't decided yet whether he wants to go through with the surgery. Although he may get monetary compensation from his employer, George would prefer to have unimpaired vision instead. He wishes he had refused to do the work under those unsafe conditions, as he knew he should have. Hindsight is often 20/20.

Protection of Children's Eyesight

Children must be taught how to handle dangerous objects. Scissors, sticks, pencils, and knives should never be carried with the ends pointed up or toward someone else, since a child, or anyone for that matter, could fall and poke their own or someone else's eye. The dangers of beebee guns, fireworks, darts, bows and arrows, and so forth should be emphasized. Unsupervised play with dangerous objects is asking for trouble. Similarly, toys should be chosen with common sense to avoid sharp points or materials that may shatter. Preventive medicine is the most effective kind.

These cautions are not to mean that you should not participate in the various activities discussed, only that you should be properly protected. If you are still injured, however, please do not be embarrassed or hesitate to call an ophthalmologist under any circumstances.

PREVENTIVE MAINTENANCE: FREQUENTLY ASKED QUESTIONS

Can I Wear Out My Eyes If I Read Too Much?

Your eyes were made to be used and they do not wear out by using them, for example, when reading. The pain around your eyes that may be noticed when you do excessive close work is often related to the muscles on the outside of your eyes that move your eyes into the proper position. Sometimes a brief rest is enough to relieve the problem, just as resting your legs after a long run relieves that pain. The nerves and other parts inside your eyes are not harmed by close work.

Good light for reading is important mainly because it makes reading easier. Although it does not harm your eyes to read in dim light, it does make it harder and your eyes may become tired more quickly. The reason for this is probably that the muscles on the outside of your eyes keep trying to get your eyes into a more favorable position to obtain the most light. The muscles don't wear out, though, anymore than a long distance runner's leg muscles do. They just become tired with this type of excessive use. This sort of fatigue is not something that can be prevented by exercising your eyes. They get plenty of exercise in everyday use. The normal strength of the muscles that move your eyes is far more than what is needed. Good light also enables you to see greater detail and color.

Sometimes after reading for a period of time the print appears to blur. Assuming that you have proper glasses (if needed), this problem can sometimes be relieved by resting your eyes periodically for short intervals. For example, looking up from the page and gazing off into the distance for a few seconds may be enough rest to allow you to begin reading again without difficulty.

Children can read material much closer to their eyes than adults since they are able to provide more focusing power. Because it is not uncomfortable for them to do so, many children hold books quite close to their eyes since everything then appears larger. Unless this is a symptom of something more serious, it is not by itself harmful. As children grow older they find it more comfortable to hold the reading material at a more usual distance. An examination by an ophthalmologist can determine if there is another reason for the child to be holding the material so close.

The same is true for watching television. Some color television sets manufactured before 1968 may have excessive x-ray emissions and you should sit at least three feet away from these sets for that reason. Television sets should be kept in focus and there should be background lighting in the room in order to reduce eye fatigue.

What Vitamins Can I Take to Improve My Eyesight?

Since your eyes are part of your body, those health measures that are basically good for your body are also good for your eyes and include such elementary things as a good diet, enough sleep and exercise, and proper hygiene. There is no specific diet that is most helpful for your eyes. It is true that vitamin A (carrots being a good source), is a critical material for good visual function, but you should remember that a very small amount of it is needed since it is used over and over by the body. (In normally functioning people, large amounts are stored in other areas of the body for replacement purposes when molecules are damaged.) Therefore, large quantities of carrots will not inevitably foster better vision. And too much of a good thing can be equally unhealthy. Excessive amounts of vitamin A can cause swelling of the brain and nerves of the eye which can cause double vision, among other things. Excessive amounts of vitamin D can cause deposits of calcium on and in the cornea, which reduces vision.

Of course, there are definite preventive steps to take. Excessive use of alcohol should be avoided because of its toxic effect on cellular function. Smoking can cause eye irritation and indirectly cause other problems by its effect on the heart, lungs, and blood vessels. Problems that affect blood vessels, such as high blood pressure and being overweight, also affect the eyes since they receive nourishment from blood vessels. Your family physician can advise you further about controlling these problems.

What About Sleep and Exercise?

Most people need about eight hours of sleep per night, but some people need much less and others a little more. Burning and redness of the eyes, particularly when you have not had enough sleep, are frequently relieved by a good night's sleep. Exercise is important because keeping your heart and lungs in good condition means that they can pump blood with oxygen and other nutrients to your eyes more effectively. However, this doesn't mean that you need to run 20 miles a day to have healthy eyes. Your family physician can advise you about what is appropriate exercise for your age and condition. Please note that any planned exercise after surgery on your eyes should be discussed with your ophthalmologist first.

What About Eyewashes?

Keeping your hair, scalp, face, and fingers clean is particularly important as far as your eyes are concerned. For infants, children, and even adults, "baby shampoo" is specially formulated so that it is less irritating if some gets underneath the eyelids. You can use a cotton-tipped applicator dipped in baby shampoo to scrub the lids and lashes, particularly along the area where the lashes come out of the lids (see Fig. 12). This will remove most debris and keep the pores from becoming clogged. This also reduces the chances of infection since some bacteria trapped in clogged pores grow quite well. A variety of products are available as eyewash solutions, for example, boric acid eyewash. Generally these are not necessary since splashing plain water on your eyes with the lids open is sufficient, but they are usually not harmful.

What Causes Allergies?

Many people are allergic to various commonly used items. To be allergic in medical terms means that specific chemical reactions occur in the body that are noticed as irritation, redness, or swelling. Not everyone exposed to the same agent will have an allergic reaction. Only people who are allergic to the agent will react adversely. People can also become allergic to substances that previously gave

FIGURE 12. Lid Scrubs. A cotton-tipped applicator and baby shampoo can be used. Be sure to rub vigorously enough along the area where the eyelashes enter the eyelid.

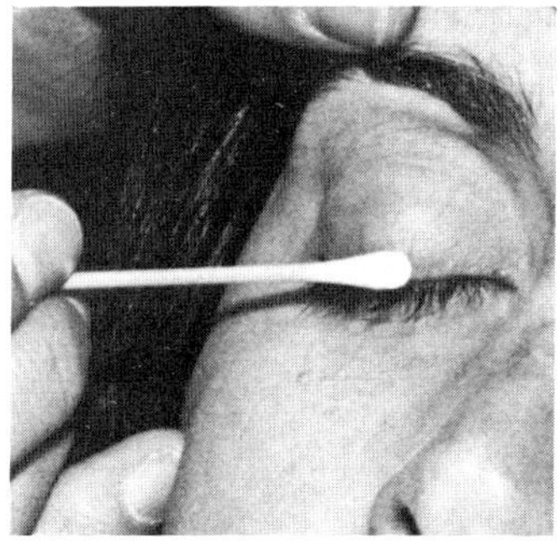

them no problem. Such items include soaps, cosmetics, powders, and sprays. Perfumes in soaps can cause an allergic reaction and various laundry soaps that towels have been washed in can also cause such a reaction. Foods and seasonal pollens and weeds are other possible allergy-causing agents, known as *allergens.* Many types of tape such as paper or adhesive tape, preservatives in drops, and even facial tissues have been known to cause severe allergic reactions. In short, it may be quite difficult sometimes to isolate the particular item that is causing the problem in a given individual, but the above-listed items can be a starting point.

Cosmetics can also cause problems because the bottle can become contaminated and infections may then occur. Your skin normally has bacteria on it and the applicator brush can transfer these bacteria to the bottle or container where they can multiply. Cosmetics generally cause more of a problem from irritation and infection than from true allergy. These problems can be minimized by keeping the eyelids and lashes clean, as previously described, and by applying makeup away from the area where the lashes come out of the lid. For example, applying makeup to the tips of the lashes is better than applying it to the lashes closer to the skin of the lids. If you do have an infection, it is best to discard the old makeup and buy fresh preparations to use after the infection is resolved. This helps prevent re-infection.

Sometimes just trying to keep the lids clean is not the best solution, as this case shows:

Case 6

Donna R. came to me complaining of pain, redness, and mattering of her eyes. I thought she had conjunctivitis and prescribed antibiotic drops for her to use. In addition, I suggested she stop wearing her eye makeup. The problem resolved and a week later she came back with the same problem. She was wearing makeup again, and was using the same makeup container. I thought she either didn't recall or didn't believe me when I said that she should use fresh makeup if she was going to use it at all. She finally admitted that she just hadn't wanted to spend the money for new makeup. After several more episodes I suggested she simply stop using makeup around her eyes. She was still reluctant; however, when her boyfriend told her he really preferred the way she looked without the makeup, but had been afraid to say so, everyone was happy.

Obviously, there is a range of what is good for each person and strict guidelines covering all possible occurrences are not feasible. Your ophthalmologist and family physician should be consulted for more information on preventive eye care.

CHAPTER 2

Understanding Your Vision Problem

A BRIEF HISTORY OF THE EYEGLASSES

The use of lenses to observe the stars seems to have been first mentioned in writings about a Chinese emperor who lived in 2283 B.C. In the time of Confucius (551–479 B.C.) lenses were probably used for sunglasses. There is no substantial evidence that they were used for visual purposes. Marco Polo reported that during his time in China between 1271 and 1295 A.D. elderly Chinese used convex lenses to help them read, although it is not clear where these lenses originated.

The first time a set of lenses was mounted on a frame to form a pair of spectacles seems to have been in Venice between 1270 and 1280. Lenses were originally scarce and expensive, but after the invention of printing convex lenses became more widely used as reading glasses. The first use of concave lenses for correction of nearsightedness (myopia) was about 1425. One of the earliest pictures of eyeglasses in use is in Raphael's portrait of Pope Leo X in 1517. The use of cylindrical lenses for the correction of astigmatism did not occur until about 1827. Bifocals were invented by Benjamin

Franklin in 1775 and trifocals were first used in 1826. Contact lenses are quite new—they were not widely used until about 30 years ago.

DETERMINING NEED FOR EYEGLASSES: REFRACTIVE ERROR

The primary indication for prescribing eyeglasses is a need to change the position on which light is focused. Ideally, light is focused precisely on the nerves in the back of the eye. This area, the *retina,* is analogous to film in a camera and is about equal in thickness.

Many factors determine where incoming light is focused. If these factors are in perfect balance, light is focused precisely on the retina and eyeglasses are not needed. If any of these factors is even slightly out of balance in relation to the other factors, light is focused slightly in front of or in back of the retina, and the individual is said to have a *refractive error.* These factors mainly include the front-to-back length of the eye, the power of the cornea, and the power of the lens inside the eye.

Although the length of each person's eyeball from front to back is about the same, they are not all *exactly* the same. The cornea, which is the clear, outer curved front surface of the eye, overlies the iris, which is the colored part. The shape of the cornea primarily determines the amount of power it has available for focusing light. Ideally, it is shaped almost like a hemisphere, that is, like one-half of a basketball. If the cornea is a little steeper in the vertical meridian than in the horizontal meridian, for example, it has more power in one direction than another and then all incoming light is not properly focused. This condition is called *astigmatism.* To understand astigmatism, one might think of a side view of a football or an egg as an exaggerated example of the corneal shape. The curvature of these objects is not uniformly steep in all directions as is the basketball's. The actual difference in curvature radius of different meridians in people with astigmatism is usually one millimeter or less, but this is enough of a difference to cause considerable distortion and a diminishment of visual acuity (see Fig. 13). Thus, astigmatism is, in the common case, basically an abnormal curvature of the cornea. Normally, the power of the cornea does not change significantly,

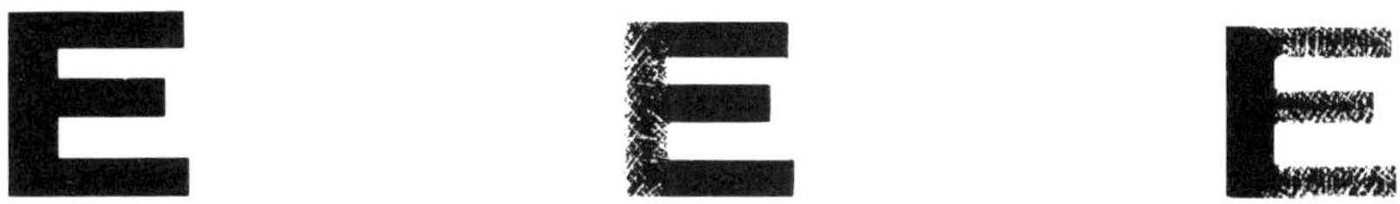

FIGURE 13. Astigmatic view. If the cornea has more power in one direction such as up and down, than another, such as right to left, all parts of an object will not be completely in focus at the same time. For example, either the vertical line (c) or the horizontal lines (b) of the letter E will be in focus at one time. In a normal person without astigmatism (a), both the vertical and horizontal lines would be in proper focus at the same time.

and the eye problem is not as serious as it may sound. Individuals with slight astigmatism may not require eyeglasses.

The lens, which is inside the eye, can, however, change its shape to a certain degree, and it is this ability of the lens to alter its shape and thus its power that enables us to focus both far away and close up. The cornea and the lens are living tissues. During childhood and adolescence they are growing and changing, just as the length of your eye and your entire body does during these growth periods. This is why eyeglasses often need to be changed frequently over these developmental periods. This does *not* mean that your eyes are getting worse. As long as the nerves respond normally when light is properly focused on them, even if different lenses are needed to do this, it is *not* proper to say that the eyes are deteriorating.

The real problem is for the power of the cornea and the power of the lens to be appropriate for the length of the eye, at all stages of growth. It is amazing that these factors are ever exactly synchronized, but frequently they are, and those people generally do not need glasses, at least not until they need reading glasses (this problem is discussed later in the chapter). For many people, however, these three crucial factors are not precisely right and glasses are used to correct these small variations. Usually when growth stops, the prescription for eyeglasses stabilizes. Hereditary and other unknown causes are thought to influence these ratios.

There are a number of other factors that also contribute to a refractive error, but they do not usually contribute as much to the condition as the ones just discussed. Some of these additional factors would be the distance between the cornea and the lens; the state of hydration of the cornea, that is, whether it is swollen; and astigmatism that is also present in the lens.

DISTANCE VISION PROBLEMS: CAUSES AND CORRECTION

People who can see objects close up without glasses but who need them to see in the distance are called *nearsighted* or *myopic.* They have eyeglass lenses that are concave and are called minus-power (−) lenses. These lenses are thinner in the center than they are at the edges. A *farsighted* person can see objects in the distance without glasses, but needs them to see objects that are close. These people are called *hyperopic* and wear convex lenses that are called plus-power (+) lenses. Plus-power lenses are also used in reading glasses and after cataract extraction. Plus lenses are thicker in the center than they are at the edges. Higher power lenses of either type are thicker, as are larger lenses of the same power. Astigmatism can occur in myopic or hyperopic individuals and is corrected with cylindrical lenses. These lenses have their power in only one orientation, which is called the axis. Safety glasses for industrial and athletic use may be thicker than glasses worn for everyday use.

A normal person does not need additional plus or minus power to see far away. They do, however, need plus power to see close up. In people under the age of 45 this plus power can be easily supplied by changing the shape of the lens inside the eye. The younger a person is, the more elastic the lens is, and so the more easily this needed plus power can be provided.

Children are usually somewhat hyperopic. This means that they need plus power to see far away and even more plus power to see close up. The normal lens inside a child's eye is so elastic that a child can easily supply 5 to 10 times as much plus power as is needed. Thus, their hyperopia does not cause a problem. Glasses are, therefore, not generally prescribed for small amounts of hyperopia in children, if there is no other problem. As the eyeball increases in length along with growth of the whole body, the eye becomes more myopic. This accounts for the common occurrence of myopic individuals first needing glasses around their teenage years. Such individuals were generally not as hyperopic when they were younger as those individuals who end up not needing glasses (emmetropes) in their teenage years.

There is a rare form of myopia that rapidly increases, and to a great degree. This has to do with the length of the eye increasing excessively, probably because of a weakness of the supporting tissue. Individuals with this condition may also have other problems with their eyes and other parts of their body. The condition is called *pathologic* or *malignant myopia* and may require a special ophthalmological examination.

Older individuals who are hyperopic may notice as they get older that they can see more clearly in the distance without glasses than they could previously. This is caused by the fact that sometimes as the lens inside the eye gets older, its power changes in such a way as to make the refractive error more myopic. Adding this new myopia to the original hyperopia may make the individual emmetropic, at least for a while.

Pregnancy can also affect the refractive error. Usually the situation reverts back to the original state a few months after delivery. Fluid retention can cause swelling, and thus shape and power change in the lens.

NEAR VISION PROBLEMS: CAUSES AND CORRECTION

About the age of 45 everyone notices that reading material is clearer when held slightly farther away than they have been used to. Those people who are nearsighted (myopic), that is, people who need glasses primarily to see things far away, also notice that reading material can still remain clear if they take off their glasses. This is all part of a normal and gradual process that is ongoing from birth. It continues even after these changes are first noted, so that eventually a person finds that his arms are too short to hold reading material the proper distance for it to remain clear. At this time reading glasses are prescribed.

For people who have never worn glasses, these changes can be quite discomforting psychologically. It should be remembered that this is a normal process and that there would be something wrong if it didn't happen. One should also realize that he is *not* going blind and that changing the power of the reading glasses in a few years does *not* mean his eyes are getting weaker. What counts is that there doesn't seem to be any way to change this process. It is the same for people in all societies and for all classes in any one society. The following case shows how psychological support can be given:

Case 7

Wilma S. was a 44-year-old secretary who was having trouble reading the telephone book. She was afraid her problem was quite serious since she thought reading glasses and bifocals were for people over age 60. It turned out that she did need reading glasses. She received them on her forty-fifth birthday, just in time to read her birthday card from her husband. The card reassured her that he still loved her even though she needed reading glasses.

This process, called *presbyopia,* seems to be related to the same biological clock that determines, for example, when a normal baby begins to walk and when puberty occurs. These events happen to all normal people within a relatively short timespan and are almost predictable by age alone. Obviously there are people who fall at either end of the age range, but it would be most unusual for a child to walk as early as three months or for puberty to be delayed until age 30. This is also true for presbyopia. Everyone within a few years on either side of age 45 finds reading glasses helpful.

Since this process is continuous, everyone will need to have their reading glasses changed about three or four times between the time they first get them and age 60 or 65. This too is normal and there is no way to change it. It does not mean that a person's eyes are getting weaker. Whether he tries to avoid wearing reading glasses or whether he wears them all the time does not affect the rate of progression. The same is true for whether one reads more or less than he used to. It does no good to try to be a stoic and avoid getting a different power when that would be more comfortable. On the other hand, using glasses of a higher power than needed can also cause problems, as we shall soon discover.

Some individuals much younger than age 45 complain of print appearing blurred after reading for long periods of time. Sometimes these individuals have a small refractive error, for example, a small astigmatic error. Correcting this error with proper glasses may relieve the problem. Other people find that simply allowing the eyes to rest will relieve the problem. Such rest periods may consist of simply glancing off in the distance, such as out the window or to the end of the room for a few minutes every half hour or so. As one gets closer to the age of 45, he or she will notice that it takes a few seconds longer than it did previously for objects to come into focus. This is particularly noticeable when looking in the distance after reading for a long period and vice versa. This is normal and is related to the same problem of presbyopia. Various medications, such as anti-intestinal spasm drugs, can also cause presbyopic symptoms. Any medications being taken should be mentioned to one's doctor. In case of any question, an ophthalmologist should be consulted.

The reason why presbyopia develops is related to the way in which the lens inside the eye lives and develops. A simplified explanation can be given. The lens is made of the same type of cells that skin is originally made from; however, it is inside-out. In the case of the skin, new cells are made at the deeper levels and are pushed to the surface. The cells on the surface are rubbed away by friction with things that are touched, or washed away in a bath. This is normal. In the case of the lens, the new cells are on the outside and the old cells keep getting packed together more and more tightly in the center of the lens. Around the age of 45, the center of the lens is no longer as flexible as it once was and so it cannot change its shape as much as it once could. Since the lens changes its power by changing its shape, one notices that he doesn't have enough power to focus closely even though he can still see clearly far away. Changing the shape and power of the lens is called accommodating. If reading material is held slightly farther away, not as much power (*accommodation*) is needed and so one can see it more clearly at that distance, although the letters will appear smaller since they are farther away.

The question often asked is whether eye exercises will help provide extra strength to a muscle that compresses the lens; people wonder if this would provide the additional change of shape required for additional power. Unfortunately, this idea does not work because, again, the system appears to be set up inside-out. The muscle that controls the shape of the lens (called the *ciliary muscle*) is contracted and withdrawn from touching the lens and lens attachments when the lens is in the shape needed for near vision. Thus, contracting the ciliary muscle loosens the zonules that stretch the lens and suspend it in proper position. When looking in the distance, the ciliary muscle is relaxed and dropped against the lens attachment sites, thus stretching the lens. In other words, the lens naturally springs into the shape needed to see near things, if it can, and is actually stretched into a longer shape by the pressure of the *relaxed* muscle resting on the zonules to see things far away. Thus, this stretching of the lens occurs by having the ciliary muscle relax and fall against the zonules. It would not help if the ciliary muscle were stronger, since it would just be farther away from the zonules in a tighter knot when it contracts. In any case, it is not putting any pressure on the zonules when it is contracted even moderately. The real problem is that the lens does not spring back to the shape needed as it does in a younger person because the center is so thick from all the cells and cell debris that have been packed together over the previous 45 or so years—and exercises cannot change that fact. The following diagrams may help to understand this concept:

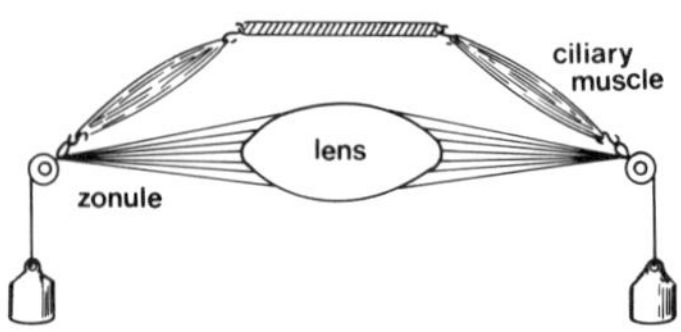

Normal person viewing distance. Ciliary muscle relaxes; zonules stretch the lens into proper shape.

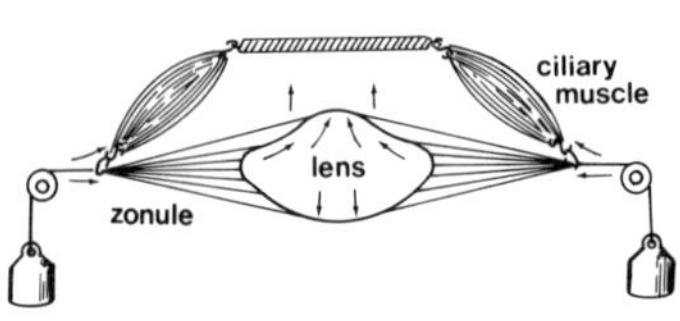

Normal person viewing near object. Ciliary muscle contracts; zonules relax allowing lens to spring into proper shape.

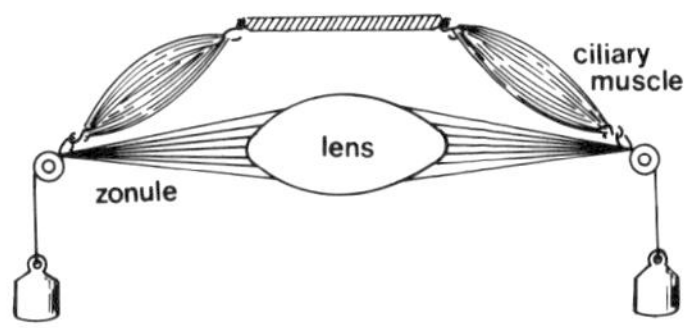

Presbyopic older person viewing near object. Lens is not elastic enough to change shape; exercise of ciliary muscle would not help.

COMMENTS ON "CORRECTING" THE PROBLEM

Glasses are worn to finely tune the process of focusing light. If you wear glasses, it does not mean that your eyes are bad or weak or inferior, anymore than needing to wear a shoe size a little larger or smaller than someone else of the same height means that your feet are weak or inferior. As long as you can walk with the right size shoe, your feet are quite satisfactory. Similarly, as long as you can see with the right glasses, your eyes are quite satisfactory. It makes no difference how well you see without glasses and it doesn't matter if they need to be changed frequently, or if they are thick or thin—your eyes are basically no better or worse than anyone else's for these differences.

Wearing glasses will correct a refractive error, but glasses will not change the refractive error itself. In this sense glasses don't cure the problem, not to the point where glasses will no longer be needed in the future. As they grow older, some people notice that they no longer need their glasses to see clearly. This is a result of a change in the power of the lens or cornea or in the axial length of the eye associated with the aging process, such as cataract formation, and doesn't have anything to do with whether a person was conscientious about always wearing his glasses. Eyes do not "improve," they simply change in condition.

People who are myopic will generally need to wear their glasses or contact lenses in order to drive safely. After the nerves of the eye have fully developed (about 10 years of age or earlier), it is really up to the individual as to whether or not the glasses or contacts are worn. After this age, the eye will not be damaged or improved by wearing or not wearing the corrective lenses. The experiences of the following two patients illustrate the range of people's preferences:

Case 8

Denise M. was a good student who was home for summer vacation. She came into my office terrified that she was losing her vision because of all the reading she was required to do. I had seen her several years before and her vision was 20/15 in each eye with glasses.

Examination revealed her vision had remained at 20/15, except that she missed two letters on that line. A slight change in her prescription would allow her to see all of the letters. Denise insisted on having the new prescription since she wanted new frames. I gave her the prescription, even though I felt it was risky to change the prescription from what she was used to for such a small change in acuity. However, Denise was very happy with the result.

Not everyone, however, is so particular.

Case 9

That same day Susan L., also a student, about the same age, came in because she needed glasses to pass the driver's license vision test. I was amazed that she didn't wear glasses all the time since her vision was so much clearer with them. Susan's response was that she preferred to see the world slightly fuzzy. Her parents look younger, for example, since she can't see the wrinkles in their faces, and everything is just "more mellow."

Exercises, special diets, undercorrection, limitation of use, and other such methods of trying to change one's refractive error have generally not been found to be of significant help. The author is not aware of any adequately controlled, proper scientific studies that suggest that these techniques are effective. There are people who contend that these techniques are, in fact, effective, but one should keep in mind the pitfalls of improper studies when evaluating whether such a method should be used. Unless these methods cause one to put off having a proper examination and thus delay the diagnosis of serious disease, such as glaucoma, they are generally harmless to the eyes, although they may be financially expensive. Recently, surgical procedures have been used to try to change a refractive error. These procedures are currently experimental and are discussed in Chapter 8.

CHOOSING AND CARING FOR EYEGLASSES

Frames

There is a variety of frames available. You should pick one in the price range you can afford in a style you like. In some cases, a particular frame style is more appropriate than another; if this is true for you, either the optician or your ophthalmologist will point out why. For example, perfectly round lenses may have a tendency to rotate if they are not mounted properly and the astigmatism axis will not be properly lined up. For people without a significant astigmatic error, this may not matter very much. Another example might be choosing too large a frame if the power of the prescription is too high. In higher powers, there are more distortions at the edges of the lenses. Some people find large metal frames with glass bifocals too heavy for them. They may slide out of position frequently and cause discomfort.

Either plastic or metal frames are acceptable. The reader should recall the earlier discussion about proper frames and lenses for hazardous endeavors. For example, frames for sports where a significant impact may occur are constructed so that the lenses will pop out *away* from the eyes and not toward them. In addition, the hinges may be more flexible so that the frames won't break.

It is quite important, however, that frames be the appropriate size for your face. The shape of the bridge of your nose, and the position of your ears may make one type of frame more suitable than another. For example, people with a flatter nasal bridge may prefer nasal supports on the sides of the nose rather than having the frame rest on the top of the nasal bridge.

Some people are allergic to certain materials that are commonly used in frames, such as nickel. A change in frame material usually resolves the problem. The allergy manifests itself by a red, swollen area where there is contact between the frame and the skin. In case of any questions, you should consult your ophthalmologist. The following case illustrates several points:

Case 10

George S. was one of those people who always looked for bargains. He was proud of how he managed to get his used car to continue running remarkably well. Thus, it was not unexpected to have him come in one day telling me what a terrific deal he got on his new glasses. He was just in time for the last day of a big sale. He proudly showed me his famous designer imported frames. However, he wasn't completely happy with the glasses because they kept sliding down his nose. In addition, his skin itched along the temples.

Examination revealed several problems. The frames were too large a size for him or for almost anyone else and were made out of a heavy metal. His were glass bifocal lenses. It was evident why these frames were on sale.

I recommended choosing a smaller frame made of plastic with plastic lenses, since this would decrease the weight of the glasses. It would also probably eliminate the skin irritation, which may have been caused by an allergy to the nickel in the frames.

When he returned sometime later after following my suggestions, George was quite happy. He decided that he would not try to cut corners with his eyeglasses in the future.

Frames must be individually adjusted and may require more than one adjustment at first. Adjustments should be available at little or no additional cost. Adjustments will be needed periodically after you initially receive your glasses, since putting them on and taking them off everyday (even if you *don't* fold the temples) causes the frames to loosen.

It is important that your frames be adjusted so that you are looking through the proper part of the lenses. If you are not looking through the correct part of the lenses or if the frames are loose and are constantly changing position, you may have headaches and pain around your eyes. This occurs because the muscles on the sides of your eyes are trying to move your eyes to compensate for an abnormal eye deviation induced by the incorrect lens position. Adjustments include not only the obvious length of the temples over the ears and the nosepieces but also such things as the tilt of the lenses, called the *pantoscopic tilt.* Properly fitted and adjusted glasses should *not* be continually sliding down your nose.

The problem of trying to repair broken frames is a real one. Unfortunately, with the large number of frequently changing colors, materials, styles, and sizes being offered it is quite difficult for an optical supply company to maintain a full inventory of all frames indefinitely. Thus, even though the lenses may be fine, new ones are sometimes needed if proper frame repairs can't be made. However, frequently it is possible to place old lenses in new similar frames, if the original frames are broken. If broken frames can't be repaired, and you want to use the old lenses, it is important that a similar frame be chosen. If the new frame is a different size or style, you may end up looking through a different part of the lens than you usually do and this can cause problems, as mentioned before.

Lenses

Lenses are made of glass or plastic. Although glass is heavier, it is not of significant difference in most prescriptions. Glass has the advantage of somewhat greater clarity and it is more resistant to scratches. All new glass lenses are either treated with heat or chemicals to make them impact resistant. They can still break, but they will not shatter if they have been treated. In higher power lenses, modifications can be made to try to reduce distortions at the edges. Such lenses are called *aspherical* or *lenticular.* The lenticular lenses have the disadvantage of a smaller visual field since the edge of the lens does not have the needed power.

Sunglasses that become darker in bright sun and lighter indoors are called *phototropic* lenses and have trade names such as Photogray. These were mentioned in Chapter 1. It should be noted that these lenses weigh a little more than regular glass lenses, and in higher power and larger frames this is sometimes a problem. They weigh more because there are tiny additional particles embedded in the glass that cause the color change and add slightly to the weight. Phototropic lenses are not available in plastic lenses or seamless bifocals.

It is possible to read the power of a lens with an instrument called a *lensometer.* This is useful for determining whether lenses have been ground correctly. Also, it is frequently possible to help find out the original prescription from damaged lenses using this instrument.

A *vertexometer* may be used to measure the distance of the lenses from the eye. The needed power is different depending on this so-called vertex distance. It usually only makes a significant difference in the higher power lenses, but it does need to be considered when contact lens power is determined.

Optical Distortions

All eyeglasses cause distortions, as does any optical instrument. However, by varying the lens curvature at different distances from the optical center, some of these distortions can be reduced. One such type of lens is called *aspherical* and is useful in reducing peripheral distortions in high-power plus lenses. Very sophisticated techniques, including computers, are used to calculate these various curvature changes and gradations. In the case of expensive camera lenses, several extra lenses are inserted to provide compensatory distortions. Yet even they are not perfect. Fortunately, most people rapidly adapt to these aberrations, as they are called.

It is important to realize that these aberrations are real and that they do exist, but that you will get used to them in a few days. If your prescription is changed, you will notice that the distortions are different from your old glasses, even though you may see more clearly. Even the same prescription in a different shape frame will cause new aberrations.

Some of these distortions can be caused by improper adjustment of your frames and frequently, just by changing the tilt or curvature of the frames, troublesome symptoms will be alleviated. If you select frames at an optician that is far from where you live and the glasses are mailed to you, it is quite important that the glasses be adjusted by an optician nearby. If you are still having problems after a week or two you should return to the person who prescribed the glasses for a re-check of the prescription and the glasses. Errors can be corrected in the first few weeks but six months later it is hard to justify regrinding the lenses at little or no charge. The following case is an example of such a problem:

Case 11

Sometimes it is quite beneficial to have your new glasses checked if there is any question. Henry T. was a famous university professor who was very precise in his work. His students, some of whom I also knew, commented on his attention to detail and how he would notice obscure mistakes. He had recently bought new glasses that were prescribed elsewhere and he was not happy with them. He tried and tried to get used to them but he felt that "something just wasn't right." Several months later, he finally came to me and a check of his eyeglass prescription and his refraction revealed that a transcription error had probably been made. It turned out that he had astigmatism in one eye that was supposed to be corrected with a cylindrical lens at axis 110 degrees. The prescription had been misread as 11 degrees (11°), so that the axis was actually 99 degrees away from the correct position. This is a rather significant deviation and it was amazing that Henry could wear the glasses at all. He was much happier after this error was corrected.

I found it hard to believe that a person like Henry would have waited so long before trying to find out if there was a problem with the glasses and not with him. Mistakes do happen, even though they are not too common.

One type of optical distortion is particularly interesting. It has to do with the fact that there is a space between the lens of the eyeglasses and the eye. One may be familiar with simple telescopes and realize that a simple Galilean telescope is composed of two lenses a particular distance apart. This distance depends on the power of the lenses used. One knows that if he looks through one end of the telescope, objects appear larger and that if he turns the telescope around and looks through it backward, objects appear smaller. It so happens that a person who is myopic (nearsighted) has the equivalent of an inverted Galilean telescope lens system when he wears his glasses. This makes objects appear smaller, but they also appear sharper since they are in proper focus. People who become more myopic in the teenage years will notice that a new eyeglass prescription of a different power may make objects look smaller, but sharper. People who are hyperopic will notice the opposite effect. This is why cataract glasses (used after cataract surgery) give more magnification than was noted by the patient before the operation, and also why a contact lens will reduce the amount of magnification in this case. The contact lens is closer to the eye and of a different power than the glasses. This is normal and is one of the aberrations that people usually adjust to rather easily, although in the higher powers it may be somewhat more difficult.

Contact lenses can also be used to correct a refractive error. For some prescriptions, because of the laws of optics, there are fewer distortions with the use of contact lenses than with eyeglasses. If this might be true in your case, your doctor may suggest them. For other prescriptions, however, it is not possible to fit a contact lens satisfactorily. Contact lenses are discussed later in this chapter.

Reading Glasses and Bifocals

Reading glasses can be prescribed as full-size lenses, half-frame lenses, or as bifocals. Convenience, cost, and personal preference are the only differences among these systems. Some people prefer two sets of glasses, using one for distance and one for near vision. However, most people, even if they don't do so for the first pair, find it more convenient to get bifocals, even if there is clear glass in the top. In certain cases of asymmetrical prescriptions for each eye or facial asymmetry, it is better to use one pair of glasses for near vision and one for distance vision instead of bifocals. These cases are rare but if it is so for you your doctor may recommend this solution.

It is important to realize how bifocals are used. The top part is used to see things far away and the bottom to see things close up. While it is true that bifocals are not the easiest thing in the world to get used to, they are certainly not the hardest, and most people manage to successfully adapt to their use. The main problem occurs when walking down steps because it is more natural to look through the lower part of the glasses; however, one really should be looking through the top part since that is the distance correction. A person may need to learn to tip his head down slightly so that he is, in fact, looking through the top part. Stairs are too far away to use the lower part, which is the part used for reading and doing close work. A similar problem happens when trying to read something that is placed at a high level such as a can label on the top shelf in a grocery store. It is necessary to tip one's head back slightly in order to look through the bottom part of the bifocals.

Some people have unusual occupational needs and require the reading correction to be placed at the top of their glasses as well. An example of this would be a house painter who might find this arrangement useful when painting the edge of the wall near the ceiling. Other occupations with special needs might include electricians and carpenters. Special needs should be discussed with one's eye doctor.

Trifocals are simply a variation on the same idea. They provide an intermediate range of clear vision and many people prefer them for such activities as playing the piano or painting at an easel, or secretarial work. The more power that the reading glasses have, the smaller the range of clear vision, so trifocals are not generally needed at first. This is also one of the reasons that most doctors try not to give stronger glasses than needed. One of my patients used another variation for other reasons:

Case 12

Rose B. came to see me at the urging of her children. They were concerned that her eyes were not normal because she had three pairs of glasses that she was continually changing back and forth.

I examined Rose and listened to her explanation of why she had three pairs of glasses. The first pair was used to drive, the second to play cards, and third to read. I asked her why she didn't just use trifocals instead and she said that she had tried them but couldn't wear them. She had arthritis in her neck and couldn't tilt her head back and forth enough to bring the lenses into the proper position. Rose was quite content to use three pairs of glasses instead and I reassured her children that Rose was not only normal, but quite perceptive.

Another reason for not prescribing stronger-than-needed bifocals is that if the power is too great, it is necessary to hold the reading material closer for it to be in focus. This means that the eyes have to turn in more (converge) to keep both eyes aligned on the print. If both eyes were not aligned and both eyes were used together, double vision would probably result. It takes additional muscular power to converge the eyes for long periods and this can lead to symptoms of eye strain. Sometimes frequent brief rests of the eyes, as discussed earlier, will manage the problem. However, in some cases optical means are needed to compensate for this problem of *convergence insufficiency*. Such techniques as decentering the optical center and the use of prisms are sometimes helpful.

The reading lens of the bifocal can be made in a number of ways. Depending on one's prescription and occupation one type may be recommended over another. Common types are the half-circle type of lens inset and the entire bottom half of the glasses made to the reading vision prescription (the line all the way across). Seamless (or no-line type) bifocals are actually a graded variation of power and have the disadvantage of having variable power, so that one is always looking around the lens trying to find the best position. They are more difficult to fit and are slightly more expensive. People who are used to conventional bifocals find them somewhat hard to get used to, but if it is a first pair there is a better chance of wearing them successfully. They are not available in phototropic-type sunglasses. The reader should ask his or her ophthalmologist or optician for more information, if desired.

It is particularly important with bifocals or trifocals that the frames be of the proper size and in proper adjustment. The level where the additional power lens is placed, that is, how high the line is, is quite important. If everything is not optimal, the glasses will not be as useful as they should be. In addition, improperly fitted or adjusted bifocals can lead to symptoms of eye fatigue, headaches, and blurred vision, among others. Sometimes it is possible to raise or lower the "line" if it is not quite right by adjusting the frames. If it remains a problem, it may be necessary to regrind the lenses.

Reading glasses are available in various drug and discount stores at markedly reduced prices. They are generally made in only one size frame, although in a variety of styles. They are available only in simple prescriptions. For some people they are adequate, but for most people they are not exactly right and can lead to distortions and headaches. Occasionally it happens that someone is so used to the distortions from incorrect glasses that he will find it difficult to get used to the correct prescription. It is far better to start out right the first time.

Cleaning Eyeglasses

Glasses need to be cleaned frequently. Once a day is not too often. A mild soap and warm water solution is usually quite adequate. Drying should be done with a soft cloth or disposable tissue so that the glasses don't get scratched. Special eyeglass cleaning solutions are also acceptable.

Do Glasses Need To Be Worn All the Time?

The question is sometimes asked whether glasses prescribed for the correction of a refractive error need to be worn all the time. There are other reasons why glasses are prescribed (other than for refractive error) that are not being discussed in this section. For refractive errors in children younger than the age of visual maturity, which is about 8 to 10 years old (see Chapter 3) it is important to have the best possible visual development and, depending on the vision problem and the prescription, it may be suggested that eyeglasses be worn constantly. For older individuals, it may not really be necessary, only more pleasant, since everything is then in focus. After the age of visual maturity, wearing or not wearing eyeglasses "constantly" will not make the vision nerves better or worse. Most people prefer seeing things in focus and thus wear their glasses most of the time, just as most people prefer to watch a movie in focus rather than out of focus. Sometimes people notice more eye strain symptoms such as headaches or pain around the eyes when eyeglasses are *not* worn, just as most people develop such symptoms from watching a movie out of focus for any period of time. This may be true because the muscles that align the eyes and change the lens power keep shifting back and forth in an attempt to provide an image more in focus. However, for many people it doesn't seem to matter and if they are past the age of visual maturity and are able to have normal vision when wearing the correct eyeglasses, it probably doesn't make too much difference if they are worn or not.

People sometimes wonder if wearing glasses will make them become dependent on them and then they will need to wear them all the time. What actually happens, however, is that people get used to seeing objects more clearly and wear the glasses more often because they prefer to see clearly. After the age of visual maturity, wearing glasses does not change the eye itself. Some people, however, find it more difficult to switch back and forth from wearing and not wearing their glasses, particularly if they have significant astigmatism or a different prescription in each eye. In such cases, a person may be more comfortable wearing glasses most of the time.

It is important to make a distinction between something causing harm or damage and something being uncomfortable. Once the visual system is mature, wearing incorrect glasses may be uncomfortable but it should not harm the eyes. This discomfort is generally relieved when the proper glasses are worn, although there may be an adaptation period. If their eyeglasses are not properly prescribed and fitted, some people rub their eyes excessively. This can lead to infections. Some people, however, get so used to wearing incorrect glasses that they prefer those glasses to ones that are more correct. In these cases, it is quite helpful and perhaps necessary to be able to examine the old glasses. These last cases, however, are rare.

Eyeglass Prescriptions

Often it is helpful to know what your old prescription was when preparing to have your eyes examined. For example, the glasses you are wearing may not be the ones you were supposed to have or thought you had, or you may be so used to a particular prescription or symmetry that changing the prescription to one equally correct may not be tolerated very easily. These records should be available at the place where you originally had the glasses or contacts made and also at the doctor's office where you received the original prescription. These offices should give you this information, frequently over the telephone, without charge or questions, if asked. Some doctors may ask you to sign a release of information form. Even cracked lenses or fragments of lenses can be useful in determining the original prescription. The lensometer discussed earlier is useful for this purpose. Thus, old or broken glasses should be brought to the examination. Many people keep a copy of their prescriptions in a safe place. A typical prescription for eyeglasses might appear as follows:

	Sphere	Cylinder	Axis	Prism	Base
OD	−3.25	+0.75	98		
OS	−3.75	+1.50	103		

Add +1.75 OU

The numbers under the headings sphere and cylinder refer to diopters of power required to neutralize the refractive error. The total number of diopters that the eye needs to provide is approximately 62. So one can see that most prescriptions are for relatively small refractive errors. The cylinder correction is for astigmatism and it has an axis designation listed in degrees. The axis determines the alignment of the principal meridian so that the power is in the right direction. A designation for "add" is the amount for a bifocal, that is, a reading eyeglass correction. It is always a sphere and almost always the same for each eye. The term OD refers to the right eye,

OS, the left eye, and OU for both, from the Latin *oculus dexter, oculus sinister,* and *oculus universal,* respectively. Prism is not used very frequently. When it is used, it is to treat a problem of the alignment of the eyes. The base designation gives the orientation of the prism.

CONTACT LENSES

It was mentioned earlier that contact lenses can be used instead of glasses to compensate for a refractive error. Some people prefer them for optical reasons. In the higher power prescriptions, or certain other problems, such as keratoconus, one has fewer distortions from the corrective lenses if contact lenses are worn. Other people like them for cosmetic reasons. Still others appreciate the fact that contact lenses do not become fogged when they come inside in cold weather. All are valid reasons for trying to wear them.

Types of Contact Lenses

Contact lenses come in essentially two varieties, hard and soft. Various modifications of these two basic types are available, such as gas-permeable and fenestrated modifications of hard lenses and continuous wear and bandage-type modifications of soft lenses. Hard contact lenses are cheaper, last longer, are somewhat easier to take care of, and are sometimes optically slightly clearer, but they are harder to fit and for some people less comfortable to wear than soft lenses.

Hard contact lenses are small pieces of plastic that are ground to fit the shape of the cornea. An instrument called a keratometer is used to take this measurement (see Fig. 14). The power is ground on the other side of the lens.

Soft contact lenses are also made of a plastic material but the meshwork is looser. Anywhere from 40 to 70 percent of the lens may be water trapped in this meshwork. For this reason, it is important that soft lenses not be allowed to dry out during storage. There are several different processes in use for manufacturing soft lenses and this accounts for the various lens parameter designations. Each manufacturer has its own code. One process involves pouring liquid plastic into molds (spin casting) and another involves the use of a

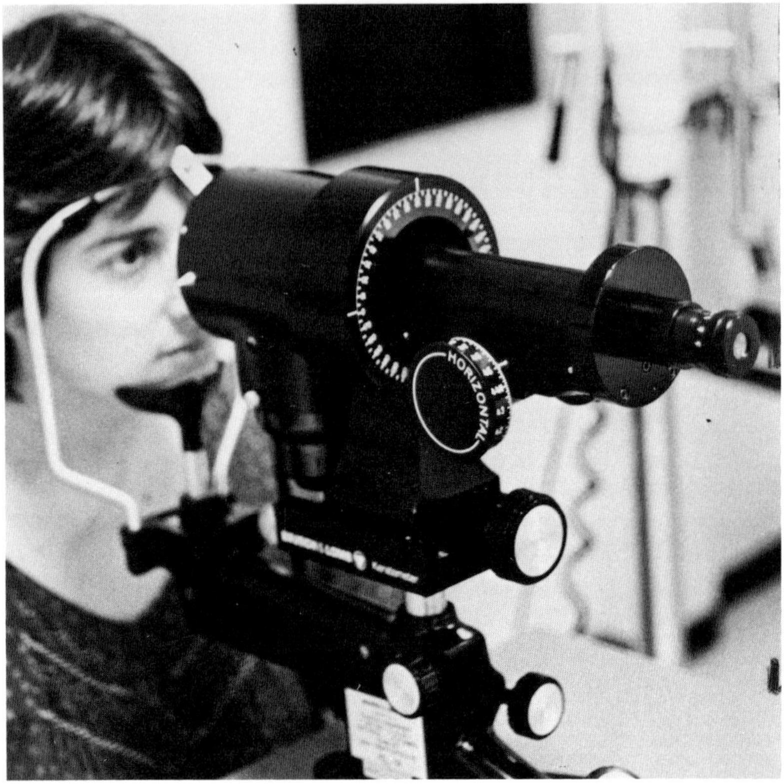

FIGURE 14. Keratometer. This instrument is used to measure the curvature of the cornea. It is helpful in fitting contact lenses, particularly the hard type, and in following any changes in curvature that contact lenses may cause. In addition, it is sometimes a helpful tool in refraction.

lathe to shape the plastic while it is hard. The lens is then placed in a solution to hydrate it to the usual water percentage.

Continuous wear lenses are soft contact lenses that are up to 70 percent water and are much more fragile. They may be recommended to people who have difficulty removing and caring for regular contact lenses, such as some elderly post-cataract-operation patients. Recently, continuous-wear soft contact lenses have become available for some myopic prescriptions. Although these patients can handle regular lenses easily, they may find continuous wear lenses more convenient. Continuous wear lenses must be used under more frequent medical supervision, since the possibility of complications is much greater. These complications include corneal ulcers and infections that can result in total loss of vision. However, they are worn successfully by many people.

Bifocal contacts are available but generally they are more difficult to fit and usually do not fit as well as conventional single-power contact lenses. Thus, they are frequently unsatisfactory. People who have successfully worn contacts before and who have low-power bifocal corrections are the more successful bifocal contact patients. As of now they are generally only available in hard lenses, although recently a bifocal soft contact lens has become available in certain powers.

Each type of lens is positioned on the tear film covering the cornea. Hard lenses normally move more than soft lenses during each blink. They are actually floating on the tear film and are held in position by surface tension. This is the type of force that makes a water droplet stick to one's finger even if the finger is upside down. Wetting agents (discussed later) are used to augment this attraction. Lenses that frequently spontaneously pop out of position may need to have the fit adjusted.

A person should have a pair of glasses to wear when the lenses are removed or lost. Since the shape of the cornea is changed somewhat by the contact lens, vision is not as clear after removing the lenses and putting on glasses. Generally after 15 to 30 minutes, much of this "spectacle blur" subsides. Hard contact lenses should not be worn more than 12 hours without a break. Soft contact lenses can be worn longer. Continuous-wear soft contact lenses may be worn for weeks to months without removal.

Insurance programs are available for replacement of lost or damaged lenses. In addition to the annual premium there is a fee for replacing the lens; however, it is less than the cost of a completely new lens.

Old Specifications

The first step in prescribing contact lenses is to have a complete eye examination. It is important to be sure that there are no other problems with the eyes and that everything appears proper so that there is a greater chance of successfully wearing the lenses. For example, a problem with frequent eye or eyelid infections may need to be resolved first. Certain allergies may make it more difficult for lenses to be worn successfully.

It is quite helpful and often quite necessary to have information about previous contact lenses one may have had or the ones that are currently being worn. This information is important for a number of reasons. Certain findings, such as the development of astigmatism, can potentially occur, and without knowing the old prescription it is hard to know if the current finding is new. Another reason is that one may be so used to one particular prescription that it is difficult to get used to another equally or even more correct one. It is also helpful to know what has been found to be unsuccessful so that the same mistakes are not made again.

This information should be available from the place where the original lenses were obtained. Generally a telephone call or letter is all that is needed and most doctors and opticians do not hesitate to give this information. It can be sent to the patient, or more often, directly to the new doctor's office. Specifically, the following should be requested:

1. Previous eyeglass prescription and vision.
2. Previous keratometer readings.
3. Previous lens specifications including type (hard or soft), manufacturer (if soft), base curve, diameter, and power.
4. Any other relevant information, such as modifications performed.

If a person has been wearing contact lenses and needs to be fitted for new lenses or glasses and old information is not available, it is necessary to allow the cornea to assume a stable shape. This can take several weeks or even months; however, six weeks is about average. Sometimes this is necessary even if all old information is available, as in the case of some types of discomfort and fitting problems or changes in certain measurements.

Care of Contact Lenses

Solutions. Many solutions are available for use with contact lenses. With very few exceptions, a solution intended for use with a hard lens should not be used with a soft lens and vice versa. All of the solutions are designed for one or more of the following uses: cleaning, sterilizing, soaking (storing), or wetting. Sometimes a solution can be used for more than one category; these are called *combination solutions*. There are several main manufacturers, each with their own trade names. New manufacturers for these products enter the market from time to time, so it is best to follow your doctor's recommendation so as to have up-to-date information on available products.

Basic Hygiene. It is quite important to wash your hands thoroughly before handling either type of lens. Be sure to rinse all of the soap off your hands. If you have long fingernails you should be careful not to scratch the lens or your eye. Although most women don't like to do it, it is best not wear eye makeup, such as mascara, when you wear contact lenses. Oils and debris from unwashed hands or from makeup can bind to the lenses and make adequate cleaning difficult or impossible. If you must use makeup, you may find it possible to do so if you insert your lenses before applying the makeup and remove the makeup before taking the lenses out.

Guidelines for Inserting Lenses. Insert or remove lenses in a place where the danger of the lenses falling on the floor is reduced. A counter with a clean towel on it is one good way. If near a sink, be sure the drain is closed so that the lenses don't go down the drain accidentally while cleaning them. Hard contact lenses are usually slightly tinted so that they are easier to find if, for example, they drop on the floor. However, the color is not so intense that it changes the apparent color of your eyes, nor is it enough to act in place of sunglasses. One of the lenses may also be marked to help differentiate right from left. If it does fall, the lens should be inspected before insertion to be sure the edge is not cracked, chipped, or torn.

General Care Guidelines. Never put contact lenses in your mouth, since they can be scratched and the bacteria and enzymes in your saliva can cause damage to your eye. Only prepared solutions should be used, especially for soft lenses. Soft lens solutions are manufactured to what is called a certain *tonicity*. Tonicity refers to very small amounts of chemicals dissolved in the water to balance the tonicity of the soft lens itself, which is in turn balanced to human tears. Plain water does not match this tonicity and may have other impurities that can become embedded in the lens and cause damage to your eye. This is not as much of a problem with hard lenses since water is not part of the lens construction.

Contact Lens Solutions and Long-term Care

Hard lens cleaning solutions are for removing eyelid secretions, tear evaporation residues, and other debris from the lenses. There are stronger cleaning solutions for hard lenses that are used less often than the ones for daily care. Hard lenses can be mechanically buffed and polished by your doctor or by many opticians when the lenses become particularly coated with debris. This polishing should be done every 6 to 12 months, or as recommended by your doctor. Some scratches may even be removed and the edges smoothed.

In addition to the daily cleaning solution designed for soft lenses, some types of soft lenses also require periodic use of a special cleaner that contains an enzyme. Some soft lenses, however, are damaged by this enzyme solution. Check to see whether it is intended for use with your lenses. This enzyme solution is used once every week. The enzyme solution is prepared by dissolving the enzyme tablet in a specified amount of distilled water. It is important to be precise; this is the only time water that is not in a prepared solution should be used. There is usually a line on the vial telling you how high to fill the distilled water. (Distilled water is generally available in pharmacies and other locations.) Hard lenses do not require treatment with the enzyme solution. It is very important to clean the edges of all types of lenses in addition to the center. Debris tends to collect at the edge of the lens and can cause irritation when it is worn.

Hard lenses do not need to be sterilized as such since the cleaning solutions for hard lenses accomplish this step at the same time. Soft lenses must be sterilized after each cleaning, that is, every day, unless they are the continuous wear type. This is so because with soft lenses there is a tendency to have bacteria and other organisms accumulate in the water in the looser meshwork of these lenses. Two methods for sterilizing soft lenses exist, one using heat and one using solutions. The solution method is called the *cold method.* It is best not to switch from one method to the other since this reduces the longevity of the lenses. If you plan to be in places where electrical outlets are not available, then you should choose the cold method of sterilization.

Soaking solutions are for rinsing the lenses and for storage. Hard lenses can be stored dry but soft lenses must be stored in a prepared solution (that is, not plain water) or they will dry out and are then generally ruined and usually must be replaced. If a soft lens dries out, do not put it in your eye. You can try to rehydrate it, but usually you must get a new one. Thus, soft contact lenses should be kept either on your eye or in solution in the case and not, for example, on a piece of facial tissue.

Wetting solutions are applied to the lens just before insertion on the eye. These solutions allow the plastic and water of the lens to rest on the oil surface of the tears.

There are also drops that can be used on the eye with a contact lens in place. These drops can be used if a person's eye gets slightly dry. Dryness can possibly result in irritation.

Full instructions for using solutions can be found on all package inserts and should be read prior to use. It is recommended that one set of solutions by one manufacturer be chosen and consistently used. Switching solutions and sterilizing techniques, particularly with soft lenses, unless directed to do so by your doctor, generally causes problems of eye irritation and decreases the lifespan of the lenses. These solutions are widely available in drug stores and chain grocery stores. Do not use solutions other than those recommended by your doctor. This includes many solutions that may sound or are spelled almost the same. Some of these are older products that had problems of one sort or another and have been replaced by the more satisfactory, recommended solutions.

The actual technique of insertion and removal of the lens can best be demonstrated in the doctor's office when the lenses are delivered. There are a number of techniques that can be used; each person usually develops a system that works best in his or her situation. It is also important to note that the case where the lenses are kept must be kept clean as well. This is conveniently done while the lenses are being worn.

As contact lenses become older, they may warp somewhat or the edges may become nicked or scratched. There are instruments that can be used to check the specifications of contact lenses, including the various curves, power, and the edge profile. This is much easier to do for a hard type of lens. These parameters are checked and recorded when the lens is new. It is important to keep the lenses away from excessive heat to help prevent warpage and, in the case of soft lenses, drying out. (For example, do not leave the lens case on top of a radiator.)

When inserting a soft lens it is important to be sure the lens is not inside out (see Fig. 15). The edge should appear to go straight up when the lens is held on the finger, just as the edge of a cup would appear. If it is inside-out, the edge will flare out somewhat as a saucer would look. Your doctor can instruct you further and demonstrate these differences. If you put the lens on the eye inside-out it will not be as comfortable as it should be and you will notice blurry vision. Just after a soft lens is inserted there may be an air bubble under part of the lens. Blinking and closing the eye somewhat tightly will usually push the air bubble out.

Wearing Schedules

It is important to understand that there is an adjustment period when you wear contact lenses. The initial wearing schedule will be prescribed by your doctor but in general it takes a week or two for one to be able to wear contact lenses a full day without a rest. This is true for both hard and soft lenses. For this reason, you should plan to wear your contact lenses every day or almost every day. In other words, it is difficult to wear them only one or two evenings a week. This is more of a problem with hard lenses, but even soft lenses have an adaptation period.

Contact lenses should not be worn when you swim or when you are around aerosols or hair sprays. Besides the tendency for the lenses to come out while swiming, chlorine and other debris become embedded in the lenses and are difficult, if not impossible, to completely remove. Aerosols also become embedded in the lenses. If you need to spray your hair after the lenses are in, you should keep your eyes closed until the droplets have settled. Contact lenses should also not be worn in a chemistry laboratory. Fumes can also become embedded in the lens and if an accident should happen, proper rinsing

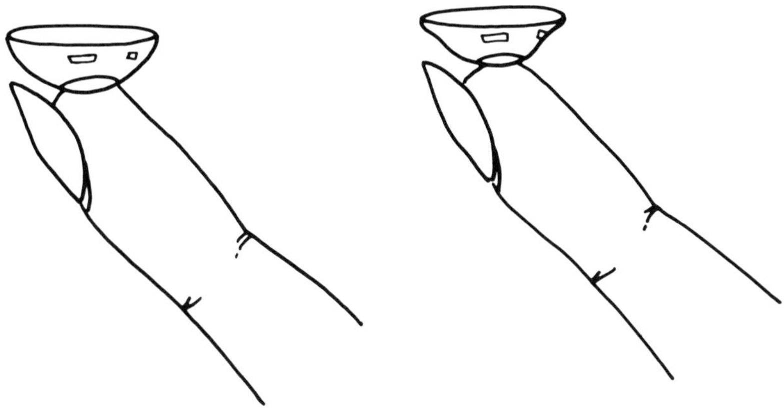

FIGURE 15. Soft contact lens. It is important to be sure the lens is not inside-out. In the proper configuration, the edges go straight up. If the lens is inside-out the edges flare out.

of the eye is not possible with a lens in place, and it may not be possible to remove it without special techniques.

Problems with Contact Lenses

There are several reasons why some people cannot wear or have difficulty wearing contact lenses. Some of these reasons are possible to predict in advance but others can only be discovered by actually trying them. Problems arising from optical causes can often be predicted. For example, sometimes a person has too much astigmatism to wear a lens successfully, although there are newer lenses that are more successful in treating this problem than were available in the past. Another such problem would be a person who is nearsighted (myopic), about 40 years old, and wants to start wearing contacts for the first time. Such a person may have more trouble reading with the contacts than with glasses.

In addition to optical reasons, there are a number of other reasons why people may not be able to wear contact lenses; for example, inadequate tear secretion, too lax or too tight eyelids, or allergy to the lens material or solutions. It is important to blink completely and frequently when wearing contact lenses. This is because the cornea normally receives much of the oxygen it needs directly from the air. When a contact lens is worn this is not possible and the cornea must receive oxygen in a different way. Oxygen is normally dissolved in tears and during a blink, tears with oxygen are circulated under the lens where the oxygen can then be used by the cornea. With a soft lens, oxygen in the air can dissolve in the water of the lens itself and be available to the cornea. This is why a soft lens can be larger than a hard one and also does not move as much. After the initial adaptation period most people learn to blink properly without frequently reminding themselves. Gas-permeable lenses are made of a somewhat different plastic that allows some oxygen to pass directly through the lenses. Fenestrated lenses have very small holes in them to allow more oxygen to pass through. These holes are not easily visible and may become clogged by deposits from tears and other matter. Your doctor can discuss with you which type of lens is best in your particular case.

Sometimes people who normally wear their lenses successfully will notice that it feels like there is a dust particle under the lens. This is particularly true in smoke-filled or dusty areas. Frequently removing the lenses and cleaning them and then reinserting them will solve the problem. If it doesn't, and especially if the sensation persists after the lenses have been removed, the individual should notify his or her doctor. A person should not rub his eyes with the lenses in position. Contact lenses may also be less comfortable when a person is sick or pregnant. Corneal swelling may occur and give symptoms of blurred vision and seeing haloes around lights, or the feeling that one is looking at objects in a smoke-filled room. Other signs of possible serious trouble include excessive pain, redness, tearing, and sensitivity to light. Many of these problems occur when the lenses have been worn for too many hours without a break. Often there is a 6- to 10-hour time lag between the time the lenses have been overworn and removed and the time the symptoms develop. Consult your doctor if you encounter a problem like this.

Infections and corneal abrasions are possible complications of contact lens wear. These topics are discussed in Chapters 4 and 6.

Suffice it to say that they generally occur when proper hygiene has not been observed or when the lenses have been worn too long without a break. These problems can be quite serious and an ophthalmologist should be consulted. One should not resume wearing the lenses after such a problem until directed to do so by the doctor. It is usually necessary to gradually build up the wearing time, as when the lenses were originally received. Continuous wear lenses have a higher incidence of these complications and closer supervision is necessary when they are prescribed. Any persistent pain, tearing, or redness, or any question at all should be discussed with one's doctor. The following cases illustrate some of these problems:

Case 13

Linda L. was a cheerleader and straight-A student. She was one of the more popular women in her high school class. She wore hard contact lenses, for both optical and cosmetic reasons, for many years without problems. The night of the Senior Prom she was out all night at one party after another and fell asleep with her contact lenses still on her eyes. She awoke about eight hours later with excruciating pain in her eyes and a severe headache. She could hardly open her eyes and any light made the pain worse. She described the pain as feeling like needles jabbing her eyes.

Examination showed a moderately severe corneal abrasion in each eye. Treatment included patching each eye closed. During the three days it took for the abrasions to heal, as her hangover also cleared, she thought about what it might be like to lose her vision and was terrified. She worried that she would not be able to attend college or continue enjoying life as she had. She swore that if she recovered she would never make that mistake again.

Linda is back to normal now and wears her contacts comfortably. However, she has been quite careful not to overwear them again.

Case 14

Gayle L. was another young woman who overwore her contacts, but for a different reason. She had a moderate degree of astigmatism and wore hard contact lenses. When she removed her lenses at the end of the day, her vision with her glasses was not quite as clear as with her contacts. This spectacle blur was caused by mild swelling of her cornea after wearing the contacts. She really did not like the spectacle blur

> and so she would wear the contacts for longer periods of time than she knew she should. This led to more spectacle blur lasting a longer period of time. She would then wear the lenses even longer. One day it was a little too long, and she too had corneal abrasions.

Sometimes after people have been wearing contact lenses for a number of years the original prescription and lenses are no longer as appropriate as desired. This may occur simply because the individual is several years older and the eyes have grown slightly in that time. Generally, as mentioned earlier, it is necessary to omit wearing the lenses for a period of time until the measurements stabilize. The cornea will tend to revert toward its original configuration if it has been somewhat distorted over the years, and as any swelling subsides. Eyeglasses can be worn during this period. Since the cornea is changing its shape and thus its power, the prescription for the glasses will also be changing, so vision will not be as sharp as desired during this period. Although the glasses can be changed during this time it is not usually done unless it is a substantial change in prescription. This is because by the time the glasses have been made, the prescription may have changed again. It may take anywhere from several weeks to several months for the corneal measurements to stabilize. Six weeks is a common time period for stabilization in many people.

A properly fit contact lens should not significantly distort the cornea. The use of contact lenses to deliberately alter the shape and thus the power of the cornea is called *orthokeratology*. It has been generally used by people other than ophthalmologists. The experience of ophthalmologists has been that the results are not predictable and that the cornea may actually be converted into a less desirable shape, from which it may not recover. Decreased vision may then occur. In addition, generally after use of the contact lens has been discontinued, the cornea tends to revert to its original configuration, thus requiring the use of a "retainer lens," or glasses. This technique should therefore be termed experimental.

At one time people thought that contact lenses might eliminate the need for frequent eyeglass changes during adolescence, but it is now felt that this eye condition stabilizes anyway for most people when rapid body growth stops, and that contact lenses have no effect on this process.

It is not possible to lose the contact lens behind the eye, although it is possible for the lense to move under a lid and appear as if it has. The reason it can't do this is because there is a thin membrane called the *conjunctiva* that blocks it from doing so. The conjunctiva covers the underside of the eyelids and the white part of the eye in a continuous, connected manner. It acts as a barrier not only to contact lenses but also prevents bacteria and other debris from going behind the eyeball. In cases of severe trauma without proper protective gear, it might be possible to break this membrane and have a lens migrate behind the eye. However, in normal circumstances the lens cannot move behind the eye. Even though a soft lens may get folded in half and be under the upper lid and appear to have gone behind the eye, it really has not done so. It is usually fairly easy for an individual to reposition a lens that is out of alignment. Your ophthalmologist can discuss the technique with you.

Most people who truly want to learn to wear contact lenses can learn to insert and remove the lenses. Most people think that they will have difficulty performing such manipulations around their eyes but most do manage with some practice. This fear should not be the reason for not wearing contact lenses if one really does want them. When they are on the eyes, they basically feel like a tear drop. Remember that millions of people wear contact lenses successfully. Many people who have never worn them before learn to wear them when they are older, for example, those who have had cataract operations. Of course, the proper fit is necessary in addition to the proper motivation.

One final suggestion: It is a good idea to have a card in one's wallet or purse stating that contact lenses are worn. If one is injured, those people providing assistance can remove the lenses so that additional problems do not develop.

Recent Developments

Soft contact lenses have recently been used as a "bandage lens" to protect the cornea during healing. Newer lenses on the market can now be used in people with more astigmatism than was previously possible, and some people have successfully worn the newer soft lenses continuously for several weeks at a time (as discussed earlier). Contact lenses can also be used to cover cosmetic defects, such as absence of part of the iris or large scars through the use of special coloring material.

SPECIAL VISION PROBLEMS

Loss of Color Vision

This section contains a discussion of what enables us to see in color and loss of this ability—*color blindness.*

For our purposes, light can be considered to act as a wave. Visible light consists of wavelengths that vary in length from about 380 nm to about 760 nm. One nanometer (nm) is equal to 0.000000001 meter and one meter is approximately 39 inches. This is a very small range. Wavelengths of the same type, but either longer or shorter than those of visible light are termed ultraviolet light, infrared light, x-rays, or radio waves. The entire range of these wavelengths is called the electromagnetic spectrum.

As has been previously mentioned, light is focused onto the retina by the cornea and lens. The retina is a thin tissue, about as thick as a piece of tissue paper, containing structures called photoreceptors which activate nerves that send impulses directly to the brain. The retina lines the inside rear surface of the globe.

There are two main types of photoreceptors and they are called rods and cones, because of their shapes. Rods are more sensitive in dim light and are not sensitive to colors. They do not allow as fine discrimination as cones do and are distributed throughout the retina, except in the very center in an area called the center of the macula (or fovea). The macula is that part of the retina that is activated when you are looking directly at an object. A light wave from an object of regard passes straight through the eye to the back and comes in contact with the portion of the retina at the macula.

Cones, on the other hand, are distributed mostly in the macula, although there are some in the periphery. There are three types of cones, sensitive to blue, green, and red-yellow light. On each side of these "color peaks" there is a range of wavelengths where the cone is still sensitive, although not as strongly. Different wavelength combinations stimulate the three types of cones in different proportions and it is believed that this is how such a large range of colors is perceived by the human eye.

The cornea and the lens of the eye filter out wavelengths of light at either end of this spectrum. Thus, the rods and cones are actually sensitive to a somewhat greater range of wavelengths than those to which they are normally exposed. When people have the lens removed from their eye (cataract surgery) some of these wavelengths are no longer filtered out. The color blue, for example, appears to be much more intense to people who have had cataract surgery. Sometimes the work of an artist will be more blue after cataract surgery for the same reasons.

Cones need more light than rods to function well; they allow perception of smaller objects. Thus, in daylight, cone-shaped photoreceptors are activated more—we can see colors very easily and are able to read smaller printed material. At night, without an artifical light source, the rod-shaped receptors are activated more; thus, we do not perceive colors as well and are not able to easily read a book. Nocturnal animals have few cones in their retinas.

It should be noted that in order for a person to look at a color or any object and say what it is requires much more than a functioning eye. All the connections between the nerves in the brain that recognize and interpret the nervous impulses from the eye must also be functioning properly. The entire speech mechanism must be working satisfactorily as well.

Defective color vision is seen more often in males than in females, although it can occur in females. The reason for this is related to the hereditary transmission of this problem and is discussed in Chapter 6. People who are called color blind are generally not completely color blind. They are usually missing some of the pigment in one or more types of cone, or the pigment is abnormal, or those cones that do have pigment do not work as well as normal ones. Rarely, all the pigment of one or more types of cone is missing. Generally, only one type of cone is affected, the most common leading to a red-green deficit. These people may still be able to distinguish traffic light colors, but would have difficulty matching closely related shades of a paint color, for example. This is called *color confusion.* Even if they have little red-green color discrimination, these individuals can learn that when the top light of a traffic light is lit it means "stop" and when the bottom one is lit it means "go."

There are other reasons aside from hereditary factors for decreased color vision. Such people are said to have an acquired color vision defect. This is in contrast to one they are born with, which is known as a congenital color vision defect. An acquired color vision defect may be related to changes in the wavelengths of light that the lens inside the eye absorbs. This commonly happens as the lens ages. This leads to colors appearing differently, just as wearing tinted glasses may change the color that objects are perceived as having. Acquired color vision defects may also be related to problems with the optic nerve, for example, optic neuritis, and to problems in other parts of the eye. Many acquired color vision defects resolve when the underlying problem either clears up or at least improves.

Loss of Depth Perception

A person can have problems with depth perception (*stereopsis*). When both eyes are functioning normally, they are coordinated so that each is focused on the object of regard at the same time. In addition, both eyes should perceive the object at the same time and the areas of the brain that interpret depth perception must also be functioning normally. Depth perception arises from the fact that the two eyes are slightly separated so that each eye views the object of regard from a slightly different angle. In addition, information regarding the degree of convergence and accommodation of the eyes is used by the brain to give depth perception. People with decreased depth perception may have good vision in each eye but there may be a problem in the connections of various nerves to the brain or they may have sight in only one eye or have lost an eye.

People with normal depth perception who lose an eye as an adult have certain problems others with different causes for lack of depth perception don't have. This is because they have been accustomed to the use of both eyes. A person who loses an eye as an adult has many emotional problems to deal with in addition to decreased depth perception. A person with this problem should realize that it is normal to be depressed for a period of time and feel anxious and clumsy when trying to do tasks that require depth perception and which were easily performed before the loss. Children adapt to the loss of depth perception more easily than adults do. However, emotional problems may be significant, and the child should be given support and self-confidence so that he or she can resume a normal life and not be bothered by the teasing of other children. It is often helpful for peole who have recently lost their depth perception to talk to other people with similar problems to learn how they have found ways to compensate for them and to receive emotional support. Your doctor can help arrange such a meeting, if desired. (Prostheses are discussed in Chapter 6.)

A person with only one good eye can use many other clues to determine spatial depth. It does take time and practice, however, to begin using these other methods. Relative size is a common clue. A person learns to recognize the size of a car, for instance, when it is at different distances away. The farther away it is, the smaller it appears. The brain is able to turn this information around subconsciously and inform a person reasonably accurately how far away a car is by how small it is. This technique does not work, however, if an object of known size is not available. However, usually a car, tree, house, or other known object is available. Commercial airline pilots are generally required to have high-grade stereopsis, since landing on a runway at high speed requires considerable accuracy of depth perception and there are no known objects to use for size comparison. However, in most situations depth perception in people with one eye is good enough to allow them to drive safely.

Other clues are also useful. For example, the shadows cast by various objects and whether one object is overlying or resting in front of another may be helpful. When doing close work that requires depth perception, the angle of the light used can be adjusted to cast a shadow. Some people find that the changing shadow helps them judge the distance more accurately. The relative brightness and blurriness of objects are also helpful. A closer object appears brighter and sharper. These techniques and others are used by artists to give a two-dimensional painting the appearance of three dimensions or *perspective.*

Another clue for depth perception is motion parallax. When objects move the relative angle changes and the brain can subconsciously use this information to help a person with one eye perceive depth. Thus, it is easier for a person to judge the position of a tennis ball when it is coming toward him at an angle as opposed to coming straight at him. A tennis player with one eye can improve his game by shifting the position of his head and body from side to side to change the angle. This is particularly useful if the ball is coming directly toward him.

It is absolutely imperative to have proper eye protection when participating in games such as tennis or other potentially hazardous endeavors. Swimming can be quite a vigorous, but less potentially dangerous athletic endeavor compared with tennis or racquetball, for example, and a person with decreased depth perception may prefer it for this reason. If glasses for correction of a refractive error are not worn, many people recommend that safety eyeglasses with no power be worn all the time as added protection for an individual with one eye.

In addition, a person can make use of what is called *proprioception.* This is the ability to know where in space one's arms and hands are in relation to the rest of one's body, even with the eyes closed. Thus, if a person with only one eye and thus little depth perception tries to pour water from a pitcher into a glass, he will usually come close but not quite close enough, if he uses only visual clues. If, however, he also used proprioceptive clues, such as holding the glass in his other hand, or touching the lip of the pitcher to the edge of the glass, he can be quite accurate.

The sense of touch can also be used when going down stairs to feel the last stair to be sure it really is the last one, and when judging the height of a curb. Relative motion and shadowing changes may be helpful when approaching a curb.

A person who suddenly has only one eye also notes problems resulting from the sudden decrease in visual field. She may bump into things or people who are in the area of field loss. It is important to realize that this problem exists and that a person can compensate for it to a certain extent by turning her head more. In social situations it may be possible to sit so that the other people in the conversation are located on the side of the remaining functional eye. This reduces the amount of head-turning and makes the conversation easier. Beware, however, of people approaching from the other side, such as waiters in a restaurant.

Loss of depth perception is a particular problem when driving or crossing a street. People with this problem must consciously learn to turn their heads more to be sure they have a complete view before changing lanes in traffic. Choice of a car with large, unobstructed windows and additional side and wide-angle mirrors may be helpful. Other problems encountered in driving with one sighted eye can be compensated for in various ways. Since parallel parking is a problem, a choice of other types of parking spaces may be advisable. Attaching pieces of wire to the sides of the car may be helpful since the wires can scrape the edge of a curb, thus signifying its location. Drawing a line in the garage either on the floor or the side wall will show how far forward to drive. With a depth perception impairment, it is important not to follow a car too closely to be extra safe. Brighter headlights may be useful for night driving to allow objects to be seen at a greater distance away.

Some people find bouncing a ball off a wall a useful exercise for developing the new visual skills that are required with loss of depth perception. After some practice in everyday activities most people find the loss to be mostly an inconvenience. It is important to realize that having only one eye does not mean that it has to work twice as hard; it will not be "used up" or "wear out" faster.

The following case gives one such person's experience:

Case 15

Raymond W. was an artist who injured his left eye while woodchopping. He was not wearing protective goggles at the time. The eye was badly cut, became infected, and was removed. He was initially quite depressed over this turn of events. He worried about his future ability to earn a living. In addition, he experienced a grief reaction to the loss of his eye similar to what he might have experienced if he had lost a close friend or relative. Fortunately, his other eye was perfectly normal.

After much encouragement and discussion Raymond began to have a more optimistic outlook on life. When the swelling had subsided and he was ready to get his prosthesis, he wanted to get seven different ones, each a different color, so he could change them each day of the week. I suggested he start with one that would match his other eye.

He gradually began to overcome the handicap of decreased depth perception. He realized that variations of the same techniques that he used to make his two-dimensional landscape paintings appear three-dimensional could be used to help him judge distances. He also had some initial difficulties adapting to the decreased field of vision. When he took his girlfriend to a restaurant he learned to sit so that she was on the side of his functioning eye. This helped his conversation. On one occasion he turned suddenly and hit a waiter who was on his blind side and spilled a tray of food and water over a number of people. He apologized profusely and sketched an amusing drawing of the scene for the other people, which not only helped him out of an embarrassing situation but even ultimately increased his business when these same people bought some of his paintings.

He has now adapted so well that when other people are having similar problems I have them speak with Raymond who tells them more anecdotes about his experiences with adjusting to his handicap. In turn, I tell my patients, most of whom still have both eyes functioning normally, to wear adequate protective eye gear so as to prevent the need to speak with Raymond, except on a social level.

CHAPTER 3

Conditions of the Extraocular Muscles

AMBLYOPIA

For a variety of reasons, one eye may not develop as fast or completely as the other and so it sees less well. This condition is called *amblyopia* and the eye with the poorer vision is called the amblyopic eye. Sometimes the cause can be determined but often it is unknown why this condition occurs. The treatment, nevertheless, is still often quite effective.

The major known cause of amblyopia involves light not being properly focused on the nerves in the back of the eye. There are many reasons why light may be improperly focused: There may be an uncorrected refractive error in one eye and no refractive error in the other one. The eye with the refractive error transmits a blurrier image to the brain and the brain begins to ignore those images in favor of the clear ones. If the problem is not treated before the age of visual maturity (age 10 or earlier), the nerve connections may not develop properly and the eye with the refractive error may become permanently amblyopic. Eyeglasses may be prescribed to correct the refractive error and patching (discussed later) may also be needed. If these treatments are administered early enough (at least before the age of visual maturity), it is often possible to reverse the condition.

Another cause of improperly focused light may be the presence of a scar on the cornea of the amblyopic eye that blocks light from getting to the nerves. Amblyopia could then develop in the manner just discussed, if the problem is not treated. In some cases a corneal transplant (discussed in Chapter 4) may even be needed.

Yet another cause of improperly focused light is one eye turning in or out too much. In order to see clearly, light must be focused on the macula. If the eyes are not aligned properly, the light cannot be focused on each macula simultaneously. Thus, only one eye is used at a time. If it is usually or always the same eye, the other one may become amblyopic. If there is frequent alternation in use between the eyes, amblyopia may not develop even though the eyes remain misaligned. Treatment of misaligned eyes is discussed later in the chapter in the section on strabismus.

Thus, amblyopia develops if both eyes do not perceive objects with equal clarity, or if the images are not aligned properly. The less clear or unaligned image tends to be suppressed. This suppression of the image from the amblyopic eye eliminates the sensation of double vision. A child younger than the age of visual maturity is easily able to subconsciously suppress the image from one eye; such a child then does not have the uncomfortable sensation of double vision. If the image is suppressed, that eye and its connections in the brain do not develop properly. The term "lazy" is sometimes used for such an eye. Lazy is also sometimes used to describe a misaligned eye even though that eye may not be amblyopic. However, an adult who sees normally and then has an accident that causes one eye to turn out will then have double vision. The adult is not able to suppress the misaligned image and this problem can be disconcerting.

In order to adequately determine the need for glasses in this condition, some children may require the use of a special ointment (atropine) prior to examination, instead of drops. Your ophthalmologist can give you full instructions on its use and possible side effects and may prescribe that it be used in the morning and evening on each of the immediate three days before the appointment. This ointment prevents the child from focusing to see close objects and also dilates the pupil. These effects are similar to those of the drops, but in some children the ointment is more effective. These effects are normal. Side effects that indicate that use of the ointment should be stopped (and your ophthalmologist notified) include high fever, rash, or bizarre behavior. This ointment takes several days to completely wear off. During this period the child will have trouble seeing close objects but often is able to see distant objects as clearly as prior to use of the ointment. Sunglasses are usually needed until the dilation effect subsides.

The eye is not completely developed at birth. A baby can recognize forms and perceive light but its vision is not developed enough to see print clearly. It is possible to evaluate the vision of small children by a number of techniques, such as showing the child pictures of common objects in different sizes or using the letter E pointing in different directions. Infants' vision can also be examined by other techniques such as occluding one eye and observing if the child has a preference for one eye or the other. Retinoscopy and ophthalmoscopy (see Chapter 1) can be performed on infants and children.

The development of the optic nerves is mostly completed by age 6 or 7 and nearly fully completed around age 10 (the age of visual maturity). This point varies somewhat from individual to individual but usually occurs between age 7 and 10. Up until this age it is frequently possible to influence this development if one eye is becoming amblyopic. If glasses are needed, they are prescribed. If an opacity is present, an effort may be made to remove it. In almost all cases, however, the most useful treatment for amblyopia, even if the cause is not known, is the use of a patch to cover the better-seeing eye.

Patching is the treatment used prior to performing any surgery to straighten the eye. The patch forces the "slower" eye to be used and to develop. For patching to be effective, it is necessary to follow the instructions given by your ophthalmologist. Generally this means wearing the patch upon rising in the morning until bedtime, with "no peeking." The length of time that the patch is needed depends on many factors, such as the age of the patient, how decreased the vision is, and the individual's response to the therapy. A very young infant may need to wear an eye patch only a few days, whereas a child nearer the age of visual maturity may need the patch for several months. Intermittent patching from time to time may also be needed.

The question is often asked if the vision in the better eye will be impaired by the patch over it. Generally this is not a problem. If vision is reduced, however, it almost always responds to reverse patching, that is, patching the other eye. The patched eye is also periodically checked by the ophthalmologist. This is one reason why it is important to follow instructions and to keep appointments.

It is important to understand that the older a child gets, the harder it is to reverse amblyopia. After 10 years of age, it is almost impossible. Even if one eye sees well, it is worth the effort of trying to improve the vision in the second eye since no one knows what sort of accident or injury may happen to the better-seeing eye later in life.

A fresh adhesive patch should be applied to the eye each morning after washing the face and eyelids (see Fig. 16). Other types of patches are too easy to remove or peek around, although sometimes other techniques may be needed. Initially, children don't like a patch partly because of the patch itself, partly because other children may laugh at them, and partly because they can't see as well. Frequent encouragement is needed and a reward system may be necessary. Decorating the patch or playing pirate games are effective means of encouraging compliance. A different manufacturer can be used if an allergic reaction develops to the adhesive backing. Two common brands are Elastoplast and Opticlude (hypoallergenic). The histories of these two patients emphasize the importance of a complete examination and proper followup with amblyopia.

Case 16

Gwendolyn R. was a three-year-old who was hit around her left eye with a tennis racket. There was a mild amount of swelling and redness of the left upper lid but otherwise the eye appeared normal. Her mother, however, was concerned that there may have been bleeding inside the eye or a retinal detachment. After applying a cold compress to the lid she brought the child in to be examined.

Examination of the left eye was normal, except for the lid swelling. However, the vision in the right eye was somewhat less than normal. It turned out that mild amblyopia was present in the right

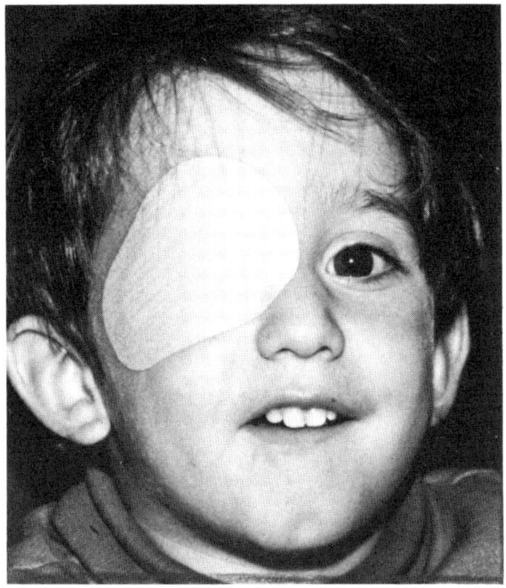

FIGURE 16. Child being treated for amblyopia. Note how the patch completely blocks light from entering the patched eye.

eye. After the left lid swelling went down, patching of the left eye was begun and a few weeks later vision was normal in the right eye. In this case, it was fortunate that both eyes were carefully examined.

Case 17

Billy C. was not so fortunate. At age six he was first noted to have reduced vision in his right eye during a vision screening examination in school. He was supposed to see an ophthalmologist for treatment; however, it was the end of the school year and Billy's family moved to a new city and he was never properly evaluated. He didn't really notice any problem since the other eye was normal.

When he was 15 years old Billy was getting ready for the Fourth of July by lighting firecrackers with his friends. He knew that this was dangerous but that made it more appealing. One of the firecrackers didn't seem to light properly so he reached for it to relight it. It exploded and he lost vision completely in his left eye.

His right eye, which had never had normal vision, was all Billy had now. It was a real tragedy that he wasn't properly evaluated and treated for amblyopia when the problem was first discovered. His presumed amblyopic eye quite possibly would have responded to patching therapy at a younger age, but now it is too late and Billy has a great handicap for the rest of his life. The dangers of fireworks and the tragedy of that incident in Billy's life are obvious.

READING PROBLEMS AND DYSLEXIA

A complete eye examination is a good place to start in the evaluation of a child with a reading or learning problem. However, quite frequently this examination shows that the child actually sees quite well and that the eyes themselves are normal or relatively normal.

The medical term for one type of reading problem is *dyslexia.* The problem in this disorder appears to be one of interpreting and understanding symbols. The problem is not in seeing or perceiving the symbols or in coordinating the eyes or whether the child is right- or left-handed. The exact cause of the problem and its precise location in the brain are not known.

It is important to realize that in this situation the problem really concerns the various parts of the brain that interpret and analyze the information that the eyes and optic nerves deliver. If the eyes and optic nerves perceive and deliver the information accurately, further evaluation and treatment of the eyes will not be of value. Treatments for this type of problem include various eye exercises and coordination evaluations. These treatments have not been scientifically shown to be effective. Your pediatrician or school teacher can suggest techniques that may be of more help.

Frequently, additional personalized help or attention in reviewing the material to be learned is effective. It would seem that this additional instruction is the real reason a child begins to do well in school. Any eye exercises or other such visual training techniques do not seem to be the true reason for any improvement that may be noted in school performance. Such programs of exercises tend to be rather expensive and time-consuming.

It should be remembered that there are other types of reading problems that are treatable. For example, emotional problems of various sorts can also cause problems in learning to read. As mentioned before, your pediatrician can evaluate the problem in terms of the child's overall development and abilities and make appropriate recommendations. If there is another real problem that can be treated, it is important not to delay the appropriate diagnosis and treatment by using unproven or ineffective techniques. The next case illustrates how problems in communication can lead to other problems.

Case 18

Jeffrey A. was having trouble learning to read. He had a complete eye examination and was found to have significant astigmatism. Glasses were prescribed which were to be worn all the time. They were not "reading glasses." However, his reading ability was still not improving. His mother wanted to start him on a course of eye exercises and other coordination techniques, but Jeffrey's pediatrician suggested talking further with his teacher.

Jeffrey's mother took the pediatrician's advice and made an appointment to see the teacher. She told the teacher that she had had Jeffrey's eyes examined and had even bought him glasses but none of this was helping. The teacher replied that she had understood that the examination was normal and no glasses were needed. The two women didn't get along very well because each had been blaming the other for Jeffrey's problems for some time.

It turned out that when Jeffrey first got his glasses, a substitute teacher was supervising the class. Jeffrey did wear his glasses; however, even though he could see more clearly, Jeffrey stopped wearing them after his friends began laughing at him and calling him "Four Eyes."

The pediatrician talked with the school principal about Jeffrey's problem: There was much more involved here than just the wearing or not wearing of eyeglasses. The dispute between the teacher and Jeffrey's mother and the additional disharmony between Jeffrey's parents were causing severe emotional problems for Jeffrey.

Jeffrey was placed in another class and given special counseling. After considerable private instruction and emotional support, Jeffrey began to read normally. It was not solely a vision problem. Actually, Jeffrey can read quite well without glasses. The need for eyeglasses was just one part of a larger problem involving the emotions of many people. Jeffrey's ability to read did not improve until these other problems were also resolved.

A child's vision should be checked annually by his pediatrician or by a screening program. With any symptom like the ones that follow, a complete eye examination should be performed by an ophthalmologist. Examples of symptoms include a child who complains of difficulty in seeing the blackboard, or for whom the letters in printed material appear to run together. Complaints of double vision, headaches, dizziness, or even nausea when doing close work or of burning or itching eyes. Sometimes these problems are caused by diseases in other areas of the body or diseases of the eye other than the need for eyeglasses. An ophthalmologic examination can help diagnose such diseases. It is a good idea for every child to have such an examination before entering school.

STRABISMUS

Strabismus means that the eyes are incorrectly aligned. One eye or both may always turn too far in or out, or it may be just an isolated occurrence. A deviating eye is sometimes called a "lazy" eye. The term lazy eye sometimes also refers to an amblyopic eye. (See the previous section.) Thus, a lazy eye may be either amblyopic or misaligned, or both.

Eyes that turn in are called *esotropic* and eyes that turn out are called *exotropic.* There are six muscles, called *extraocular muscles,* that attach to the outside of each eye. These muscles enable the eye to turn in various directions, and even to rotate slightly. In any case, it is important to have a proper eye evaluation in order to determine the cause of a misalignment, if possible. Some causes, although rare, are quite serious. For example, life-threatening tumors, which can generally be treated effectively if diagnosed early, can cause strabismus. It is important not to delay such a diagnosis by an inadequate examination or inappropriate treatment. Often no such cause can be found, but treatment, especially the one outlined below, can still be generally effective.

A complete medical eye examination must be done first. It will prove, among other things, whether there is a difference in quality of vision between the individual eyes. If so, then amblyopia is present. An eye patch may then be needed. Eyeglasses may also be needed and if so, they will be prescribed. There is one type of strabismus, called *accommodative esotropia,* that is treated by the prescribing of eyeglasses alone. The condition occurs when a person is farsighted in a certain way. In this case, glasses need to be worn all the time in order to keep the eyes straight. The power of the glasses may be decreased as the child gets older, and their use sometimes discontinued in adulthood. This is different from wearing glasses for visual clarity. Although accommodative esotropia is not rare, it is not the most common form of strabismus.

After an amblyopia has been treated in this manner, surgery is frequently needed to reposition the muscles on the outside of the eye. A muscle may be relaxed by moving it surgically a few millimeters farther back, or tightened (and thus strengthened) by removing a few millimeters of the muscle or tendon and then suturing it back in its original position. This surgery takes about one hour and is performed in a hospital. Generally, it is possible for the patient to go home the next day or even the same day. Surgery is frequently done on one muscle of each eye in order to achieve better balance, even if only one eye is deviating. Since not everyone has the same response to the same operation, a second operation is sometimes needed. This usually takes place at least six weeks after the first operation, since it takes that long for all of the swelling to subside and the more permanent result of the operation to become evident.

It usually only takes a few days after the operation for much of the swelling, redness, and irritation to subside. A doctor may or may not prescribe drops or ointments to be used during this rehabilitation period, depending on the procedure and technique used, and patient response. In any case, if there is excessive pain, redness, or discharge after the surgery or if the eyes deviate considerably more than before surgery, or if there is any other question, the doctor should be consulted without delay. Early treatment of many complications gives better results. The patient should not go swimming after strabismus surgery until the doctor gives permission to do so. Other aspects of surgical procedures are discussed in Chapter 7.

There is another form of strabismus called *pseudostrabismus.* In this condition it appears that an eye is deviating when it really is not. Young children sometimes have a flat nasal bridge and the skin covers the white part of the eye so that it looks like the eye is turned in. As the child grows, the nose generally becomes less flat and the eyes appear normal.

There is a tendency for strabismus to be inherited, so if someone in your family has had this problem all children should be examined and observed for symptoms. It is even possible to examine infants, so do not wait until the child gets older.

It is important to realize that if amblyopia exists with strabismus, it is necessary to correct the strabismus in order for any amblyopia therapy to have a permanent effect. This is why it is recommended that after any amblyopia has been corrected by the use of patching, for example, that surgery for strabismus be performed shortly thereafter. Otherwise, the amblyopia recurs and vision may be lost if the child is too old. Amblyopia is corrected before surgery in order to have a better chance of the surgery maintaining straightness of the eyes.

In children, the best results are obtained when amblyopia and strabismus are treated early, that is, before the age of visual maturity. Most people like to treat this condition before five years of age, and some may operate as early as six months of age. The following case illustrates another reason for not delaying therapy:

Case 19

Johnny J. was a young boy who had been noted by another doctor to have one eye turn in. He was three years old at the time. The doctor recommended surgery but Johnny's parents were reluctant. They kept putting it off, making excuses, and trying other remedies.

Johnny started kindergarten and after a few days he refused to go. His mother tried to find out what was wrong and called his teacher. His teacher said she was not sure what the problem was but thought he needed an eye examination, since one of his eyes was turned in.

That evening Johnny overheard his parents talking about scheduling the eye examination. He came running into the room, and burst into tears. He said that he hoped the doctor would not laugh at and make fun of his crossed eye like all the children at school.

His parents decided they would finally follow their doctor's recommendations. Johnny had surgery a few weeks later, with good results. His eyes were straight. He became somewhat of a hero at school when he spoke in great detail about his experiences in the hospital. He began looking forward to going to school and his parents were happy that the problem was resolved. They were warned that further surgery might be needed later; however, even several years later it still had not become necessary.

Adults can also have strabismus. It may occur for a number of reasons, including recurrence of a childhood strabismus, trauma, problems with some of the cranial nerves, thyroid problems, tumors, and others. For adults the results are not as good since the visual system is mature and it is harder to change. Sometimes, however, the results are satisfactory, so it is worth discussing the problem with your doctor. It is not as urgent to operate in most cases of acquired strabismus in adults. However, the sudden onset of strabismus and double vision, particularly in an adult, should be evaluated as soon as possible, since some of the causes could be life-threatening and require prompt therapy.

Other treatments for strabismus tried in the past include glasses with prisms or exercises. Generally, these techniques, when evaluated properly, have been found not to be as helpful as surgery. The reason why prisms are not as useful as one would like is that they are most helpful in only one field of vision. Since the eyes are constantly moving from one position to another, the relationship between the eyes, and thus the proper alignment of the prism, is constantly changing. For example, when looking off in the distance to the left, the left eye must rotate out and the right one must rotate in. However, when reading, both eyes must rotate in. *Orthoptics* is the name for the nonsurgical techniques used in the treatment of strabismus. Sometimes they are useful in treating a child before surgery is employed, or in cases of very small deviations. Generally, orthoptic techniques are not used as much today as in the past since the newer surgical procedures and techniques have been found to be more effective.

Exercises do serve to strengthen a muscle; however, the problem is usually not caused by muscle weakness but by an imbalance in nerve stimulation of the muscles. Exercises have generally not been found to be helpful in changing the pattern of impulses from the brain to the muscles of the eye.

New Developments

New developments are occurring in this field, as in other aspects of ophthalmology. In strabismus treatment, they mainly concern modification of the surgical procedure and the technique used, and such areas as improved suture material and needles. The newer needles, for example, are sharper and are curved to make it easier to be more accurate in their use. Usually sutures that are absorbed after a certain time period are used so that suture removal is unnecessary.

In older individuals, some doctors are using sutures that can be adjusted later on the same day that surgery is performed. This allows for somewhat more accurate placement of a repositioned muscle, as the individual is awake and looking at objects in a more normal manner when the final placement of the extraocular muscle is determined. In many cases, however, it is better to operate when the child is younger, even though adjustable sutures cannot be used.

CHAPTER 4

Conditions of the Front of the Eye

TEARING

Tears are actually composed of three major layers. The outer layer is primarily composed of oils, the middle layer is mostly water, and the inner layer is mainly a mucous layer. Various enzymes and other components are present in the tears. They are normally produced at a certain rate and drain out through openings in the upper and lower lids into the nose. If the eye becomes dry because of faster evaporation, for example, in the hot sun, normally more tears are produced. There is a number of causes of decreased tear production and dry eyes, such as extreme vitamin A deficiency, Sjogren's syndrome, and various inflammations.

One of the disadvantages of a dry climate is that more tears need to be produced faster. Frequently, people do not produce enough of the three-layer type of tear to keep up with the rate of evaporation. They then have a sensation of burning and itching that may lead to an outpouring or a sensation of outpouring of watery-type tears. A patient may also describe a gritty feeling as if an eyelash, sand, or other foreign body was in the eye. The only problem is that these tears, if produced at all, are missing one of the major layers and therefore do not work as well as they should. The person still has the burning sensation from what is believed to be an excessive amount of tears. Increased sensitivity to light and blurred vision may also be noted.

Smog is another source of similar eye irritation. Makeup, such as mascara and powders, can also cause irritation and similar symptoms, particularly if small particles fall on the eye. Normally, tears can wash these particles away, but if tear production is deficient, these particles may remain on the eye. When the eyelids blink over them, irritation can be caused. Aerosols may also cause a similar reaction. Inadequate tear production can also cause problems with contact lenses, as this case illustrates:

Case 20

Mollie A. came to me complaining that her eyes felt like they were "burning." She said the symptoms were worse when she wore her hard contact lenses. She had recently lost her lenses and was wearing new replacement ones. She thought that the new ones were not the same as the old ones, even though they were supposed to be, because they were not as comfortable.

I requested that her old records be sent to me so that I could compare the specifications of each set of lenses. It then became clear what the problem probably was. Mollie had recently moved from a city that was quite humid to one that was not nearly as humid. This move coincided with the use of her replacement lenses. After checking the lenses, the old records, and Mollie, I decided that she had decreased tear production. I recommended using soft contact lenses, advice which she followed. Mollie was then able to wear contact lenses more successfully. Even so, she occasionally needed to use a supplementary ocular lubricant designed for use with her particular lenses.

Eyes that are dry may appear red and irritated. However, it is important to realize that many other causes for a red or otherwise irritated eye exist, some of which can be quite serious. A complete eye examination can differentiate among these various causes.

Treatment

Artificial tears or tear substitutes are available as drops and provide some relief. Clearly, you cannot put a drop on your eye every time you blink and would have spread a new layer of tears across the eye. Fortunately, it is generally not necessary to use the artificial tears more than once every hour, and usually four times a day are enough. When it is more humid, drops are needed less than when the air is dry. There are a variety of preparations available; usually the word "tear" is in the brand name. Artificial tears are generally available in drug stores and supermarkets without a prescription. A good technique for inserting eyedrops is outlined in Chapter 1.

Artificial tears come in thick and thin varieties, with a few that are inbetween. Some people prefer one type over another and it is recommended that you try several brands to see which you like best. If your eyes are dry, often the first drop you put in will sting a little bit. This is normal. Wait a few minutes and apply another one. You will soon learn how often you need to use the drops to keep your eyes moist enough to reduce the symptoms. You will not completely eliminate the burning, but you should be able to control it to a certain degree.

Many people find that splashing lukewarm water on their eyes works just as well. This is more useful if the watery layer of the tears is deficient or if there are many environmental irritants. This is conveniently done when you wash your face. After all the soap is rinsed away, keep your lids open and splash water on your eyes. Some people find that a boric acid eyewash is also helpful. This is generally not much different from using an artificial tear or plain water, but it is not harmful in most cases. Some people find that using an ointment such as Lacri-Lube® before going to sleep at night is helpful in preventing excessive symptoms in the morning.

Sunglasses are sometimes helpful in reducing tear evaporation and can also be tried.

It is important to try to keep the eyes reasonably moist for several reasons in addition to the fact that it is more comfortable. When the tissues of the outside of the eye become somewhat dry, they are less able to resist infection. Recurrent episodes of conjunctivitis, for example, may ensue. Particles of makeup that accidentally drop onto the eye which would normally be rinsed away by the tears may not be rinsed away if tear production is inadequate. This can cause additional irritation and even a corneal abrasion.

A number of artificial tear preparations are available. Some of the more common ones are listed below.

Trade Name	Manufacturer	Consistency
Liquifilm Tears®	Allergan	Thin
Neo-Tears®	Barnes-Hind	Thin
Liquifilm-Forte Tears®	Allergan	Medium thick
Tears Naturale®	Alcon	Medium thick
Isoptotears®	Alcon	Thick
Lyteers®	Barnes-Hind	Thick
Adsorbotears®	Burton-Parsons	Thick
Tearisol®	Smith-Miller-Patch	Thick
Ultra-Tears®	Alcon	Very thick
Lacri-Lube®	Allergan	Ointment; use before bedtime

These preparations and others are available without a prescription in most drug stores and supermarkets.

In severe cases of decreased tear production and dry eyes it is possible for the drainage holes in the lids to get clogged. This condition is usually not reversible. (A newer treatment is discussed in the next section.) Your doctor can advise you whether such treatment is necessary.

New Developments

Recently, a long-acting preparation, called Lacrisert®, has been introduced for use in severe cases of reduced tear production. It is a small gelatinous pellet that is placed under the eyelid. It slowly dissolves over a period of about 12 hours, so that a more constant source of additional lubrication is available. It is used in more serious cases and may cause some transiently blurred vision after insertion. Your ophthalmologist can give you more information about this and other new developments.

TEAR DUCT PROBLEMS

Tears are formed in several locations. There are glands along the edges of the eyelids and also a large gland (called the *lacrimal gland*) located at the upper outer part of each orbit (see Fig. 17). Tears flow from these glands and are spread across the globe by the lids during blinking. The tears that do not evaporate flow out of the orbit through small holes (called *puncta*) in the upper and lower lids near the nose. There is one punctum in each eyelid.

FIGURE 17. Tear Duct Anatomy. The various parts of the tear drainage system. Tears are produced in the lacrimal gland and in other glands along the lid margins. They drain out the puncta in the upper and lower lids into the canaliculi, then into the sac and nasolacrimal duct into the nose. (From Frank W. Newell and Terry Ernest; *Ophthalmology: Principles and Concepts,* 3rd ed. Copyright 1974, C.V. Mosby, St. Louis, p. 43.)

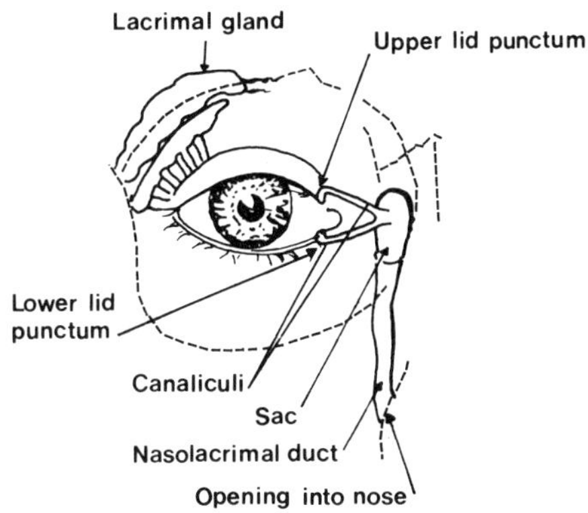

The tears flow through the puncta into small tubes called *canaliculi.* The canaliculus from the upper lid and the one from the lower lid combine to form a common canaliculus that empties into the nose. Here the tears are mixed with nasal secretions which are then either absorbed into the bloodstream, blown out, or swallowed.

This anatomic relationship helps explain why during excessive tearing people also notice that they have greater nasal secretions. It also explains why people commonly taste eye drops (at least those that have a taste) several minutes after application to the eyes.

Problems can occur with any part of this system. The punctum may be closed by scarring after an injury, for example, or it may not be properly aligned if the lids are rotated too far in (*entropion*) or out (*ectropion*), or it may never have formed properly in the first place. People with this problem may notice that their tears actually drain over the lower eyelid onto the cheek. For people who do not produce enough tears, the punctum is sometimes intentionally plugged to cause those tears that *are* produced to remain on the surface of the eye for a longer period of time. The canaliculus may also be scarred from an injury or infection, with a similar effect noted.

Problems in Infants

A somewhat common problem in babies is that the opening from the common canaliculus into the nose is closed by a very thin piece of tissue. The parents notice excessive tearing and usually pus, since the closed space tends to be a good place for bacteria to grow. Frequently, this piece of tissue blocking the opening is reabsorbed, as it normally is before birth, and the baby will then be normal. However, if this has not happened in the first 6 to 12 months of life, a small probe can be inserted through the lid and pushed through this thin tissue to make an opening. A solution is then often irrigated through to check whether the passage is really open and to flush out any residual debris. This is a fairly simple procedure and generally is effective the first time, but sometimes the hole does not stay open and another attempt at probing is needed. Probing is usually done under general anesthesia, but is sometimes done in an office. It is generally thought best to wait at least six months before probing again because the block often opens by itself and probing is then not needed. In addition, the baby is older and therefore better able to tolerate the anesthetic. Furthermore, the tissues are larger and there is less risk of creating what is called a "false passage."

If there is an infection, drops may be prescribed to try to curb it; however; usually it is not completely controlled by drops. Such an infection does not generally cause any lasting problem, but if allowed to persist for years it could cause scarring, which would lead to tears flowing over the lids and other problems. Frequently, only one eye is affected. Massaging the area in an attempt to open the blocked canaliculus is sometimes effective, but more often it doesn't really seem to make much difference.

Problems in Adults

In older people, the canaliculus (or any other part of the system) may not be functioning well, either from injury, scarring, or other causes, and tears flow onto the cheek. In these cases it is often possible to create an entirely new passage into the nose. Such a procedure is called a *dacryocystorhinoscopy,* or DCR. This is a more major procedure than probing;, here too the passage may not remain open and the surgery may have to be repeated. A DCR is always performed in an operating room. Sometimes before it is done, x-ray studies are made with injection into the punctum to better localize the obstruction.

In cases of trauma to a canaliculus, it is often not possible to align the ends of a cut canaliculus, although an attempt is usually made. It should be noted, however, that one functioning canaliculus is often enough to prevent tear overflow. Thus, the upper canaliculus may be intact and function well enough to provide normal tear flow, even if the lower one is damaged.

EYELID MALFUNCTION AND MALFORMATION

The eyelids are vital for proper functioning of the eyes. They serve a number of purposes and are more complex than one might think. First, they provide a very important protective mechanism called the *blink reflex.* This reflex is not instantaneous, but is frequently fast enough to prevent or reduce damage to the eyeball. Another part of this reflex is called Bell's phenomenon, which is noted as the eyelids are closing. As they close, the eyeball itself rotates up so that the front part of the eye is not exposed, even though the lids are still partially open. This is a normal additional protective mechanism.

Another function of the lids is to distribute the tear film evenly across the front of the eyes. This is accomplished through the normal blinking action. Tears exit from the surface of the eye through small openings on the upper and lower lids near the nose, as discussed in the previous section. The lids also have glands in them that secrete important components of the tear film itself.

Problems with the eyelids can occur in any of these areas. An eyelid may droop too much (called *ptosis*), thus blocking vision. There may be a problem with a muscle in the lid, or a problem with the nerves that stimulate the muscles. Frequently, such a problem can be corrected by a surgical procedure that tightens the muscle. Or, if it is a problem with the nerves, a drug can sometimes be used to stimulate them. Other causes of ptosis include problems with blood vessels and tumors. The sudden onset of ptosis should be considered an emergency.

Excessively Loose or Tight Lids

In older individuals the skin of the lids may be lax, which can lead to a baggy appearance. Surgical repair may be possible. Baggy lids may also be indicative of other medical problems, such as kidney disease or an allergy.

The opposite problem can also happen, that is, the lid can be too tight and not adequately cover the eye. This can lead to drying of the front part of the eye, which leads to a variety of problems, including infection and decreased vision. Such people may appear to have bulging eyes. Again, a surgical procedure may help correct the problem; however, there may also be other medical problems associated with bulging eyes that require treatment, such as a problem with the thyroid gland, a tumor, or an infection.

The part of the eyelid adjacent to the eyeball is lined with a very thin tissue called the *conjunctiva.* This conjunctiva is a continuation of the conjunctiva that covers the white part of the eye. A variety of infections and allergic reactions can affect the conjunctiva, which can lead to irritation of the lid. Frequently, drops can help resolve the problem.

Abnormal Lid Alignment

If the lid is rotated in (*entropion*) or out too far (*ectropion*), problems can develop. For example, in the case of an entropion the lashes can cause an irritation of the front of the eye. In the case of an ectropion the conjunctiva is more exposed to the air, and this exposed conjunctiva can dry out and become infected. In either case, the tear film is not properly distributed across the front of the eye, causing drying, irritation, or infection of the eye itself. A surgical procedure may help. If the lids can be returned to their normal position so that the tear film can then be properly distributed, this type of surgery may completely resolve the problem. A part of the lid may be removed or stitches placed to strengthen and rotate a weakened area. The following case is illustrative of this problem:

Case 21

Minnie T. was a 75-year-old grandmother who came to me complaining that she could not read the letters from her grandchildren. Everytime she began to read them her eyes started stinging and she had to blink to relieve the pain.

When I saw Minnie, I noticed that her lower eyelids rotated out and that they were quite loose. She was not getting proper distribution of the tear film, so her eyes were becoming dry and causing her discomfort. Although the use of artificial tears helped somewhat, I recommended surgical repair of the lids. When this was done and artificial tears were used intermittently, Minnie was able to read easily, which made her, her grandchildren, and me happy.

If an eyelid has been damaged from trauma, the edge of the lid may not be smooth and a problem with tear distribution can occur. Surgical correction may be necessary. If the lid is not properly repaired, the patient can have problems of tearing or dryness of the eyes. In cases of trauma to the lid it is important to be certain that there has not also been a problem with the eyeball itself.

The surgical procedures described in this section generally take about one to two hours and are often performed under local anesthesia. A shell is placed over the eyeball itself to help prevent any inadvertent damage to the globe. Depending on the procedure, the stitches may remain in place for at least a week and sometimes longer.

Eyelash Problems

Some people have an extra row of lashes growing along the lid margin, or lashes that grow toward the eye instead of away from it. Sometimes it is possible to remove them and cauterize the roots so that they do not grow back.

The openings in the lids where the lashes come out can become infected. This problem is discussed in the next section on styes and chalazions.

Other Eyelid Problems

Lid twitching is a common problem, usually relieved through rest. In severe cases where the lids often suddenly close and remain closed in spasm for a long period of time, a surgical procedure may be needed to reduce the amount of nerve stimulation.

Problems with the skin on other parts of the body can also occur with the skin of the lids. For example, an allergy to a particular type or brand of soap or cosmetic may also affect the eyelids. Dandruff or scaling of the skin of the lids is another common problem. *Blepharitis* is another name for this condition. It is associated with a similar problem of the scalp. Cleansing the lids with baby shampoo and keeping the scalp clean, as described in Chapter 1, are effective treatments. Sometimes a dermatological consultation is necessary. One should be careful about applying lotions and ointments intended for the skin to the eyelids because some of these preparations may be harmful to the eye. An ophthalmologist should be consulted in case of any question.

Tumors may also occur on the lids. They are discussed in Chapter 6.

STYES AND CHALAZIA

The same process that causes a pimple to occur on your face can also occur on your eyelids. Usually one of the eyelash pores is plugged up by the normally secreted oils on your skin. Makeup, such as mascara, can also plug up these pores. In addition, makeup can become contaminated when the applicator brush transfers bacteria from your skin or lashes to the makeup jar. Bacteria then grow in the pores instead of being flushed out. These bacteria have waste products that can be irritating to the cornea and give the sensation of a foreign body in the eye. In the early stages such an infection is called a *stye.* If it is allowed to persist for weeks or months, a thickened wall can form around the pore and the material inside the pore becomes more firm and rubbery. It is then called a *chalazion.*

Hot packs are generally the most effective initial treatment. The heat leads to a greater blood flow to the area, which is beneficial in fighting the infection. It also tends to dilate the pores, which helps to drain out the bacteria and bacterial debris. Hot packs should be applied as follows: Take a towel or washcloth and place it under running hot water. Then squeeze the water out and apply to the eyelid with eyelids closed. Do not make the towel too hot or you can burn the skin. The towel should only be about as hot as you can withstand on your fingers.

You will notice after about 10 to 20 seconds that the towel becomes somewhat cooler, although it is still quite warm. When this happens, reheat the towel as described above. Reheat the towel five times per session, with about five of these sessions per day.

You may notice the pimple coming to a white point. If it breaks open by itself, let it drain and apply the hot pack. Do *not* try to pick at it or to break it open because you will just spread the bacteria around. It is possible for the bacteria to be pushed into blood vessels connecting directly with blood vessels that supply the brain. Serious infection of the brain can then occur.

You should notice considerable improvement in 1 to 2 days after hot pack treatments are begun. If the condition gets worse, let your doctor know right away. Do not use any drops or ointments unless directed to do so by him. Sometimes antibiotic drops may be prescribed.

At times a tumor resembles a chalazion. Hot packs will not resolve a tumor; however, these tumors can frequently be completely eliminated if treated early. Therefore, do not delay asking your doctor if there is any question about a possible tumor.

If adequate use of hot packs does not resolve the condition, it is sometimes necessary to make a small incision and drain the fluid. This must be done under sterile conditions to prevent further infection, but is not a major procedure if it must be done. However, it is not always successful since the lining of the cavity of a chalazion must be completely removed to prevent a recurrence, and this is not always possible. A chalazion can also recur in another location for the same reasons the first one occurred. A specimen, if possible, may be sent to a pathology laboratory to be certain the chalazion is not a tumor. The following case illustrates the importance of prompt examination and treatment:

Case 22

Jack T. was a man who had what he thought was a stye. He tried using hot compresses but they didn't really seem to make much difference. He went to his ophthalmologist, who removed the lesion and sent it to be examined under the microscope. It was lucky for Jack that he sought help without delaying too long because it turned out that the lesion was a cancer. Fortunately, the tumor was completely removed and Jack has not had any more trouble.

Frequently, people have a problem with recurrent episodes of infection. It is often possible to prevent such episodes by keeping the eyelids clean with the use of baby shampoo and cotton-tipped applicators, as discussed in Chapter 1. Eye makeup may have to be discontinued or reduced in use. When cleaning the lids it is important to rub vigorously enough along the lash line. In addition, it has been found that keeping the hair and scalp clean is helpful in preventing recurrences.

PINGUECULA AND PTERYGIUM

The thin layer of cells covering the outside of the eyeball is called the *conjunctiva,* and it is related to the same cells that form skin. When either your skin or your conjunctiva is irritated by excessive sun exposure or rubbing, for example, each reacts by thickening and forming scar tissue or a *callus.*

People who spend a lot of time outdoors in bright sun or exposed to wind or dust frequently have scar formation on their conjunctiva. It generally starts over the white part of the eye (*sclera*) next to the nose and can grow closer to the center of the cornea. When the scar is only over the sclera it is called a *pinguecula.* When it also involves the cornea it is called a *pterygium.* It may appear as a white or yellow deposit over the white part of the eye and may get redder and more irritated when one is exposed to the irritants and then regresses somewhat to the old appearance after resting.

It is generally not necessary to remove a pinguecula or a pterygium unless it starts to encroach on the visual axis where it would block light from entering the eye, or if it is irritating the lids when they are blinked, or if it is cosmetically disfiguring. The operation to excise it is relatively minor as eye surgery goes, since the pterygium is on the outside of the eye. It is usually removed under local anesthesia. One of the main problems with this condition is the tendency for recurrence.

There are two methods employed to try to prevent a recurrence. Low doses of weak radiation can be applied to the affected site during surgery and on a few occasions thereafter. The radiation used is so weak that it does not even penetrate to the inside of the eye, yet it destroys many of the cells that cause this scar tissue to form. The other method is to use a drop containing Thiotepa, which is a potent drug used to kill cells. Since it is applied in drop form and is rapidly diluted by tears, there is little danger of its affecting other cells. These drops must be freshly prepared each week and are used six times a day for six weeks, or as directed. Should the scar recur, it can be removed again. Recurrences are more frequent than one would like, but for many people this never happens.

The danger of this type of scar turning into a cancer and spreading to other parts of the body is very slight. In fact, it is not a real worry. If you wait to remove it until it is encroaching on the visual axis, recovery time will be longer because there will be swelling of the tissue around the visual axis that can lead to visual distortions. It may take several months for all of the swelling to subside and your vision to be more normal. If it is removed earlier, this is not nearly as great a problem. Since a cancer can be confused with a pinguecula or pterygium, it is important to have a proper eye examination if there is any question.

CORNEA, CORNEAL ABRASION AND CORNEAL TRANSPLANT

The *cornea* is at the front of the eye. It is a transparent tissue that lies over the colored part *(iris)* of the eye. It is about 12 millimeters in diameter and about 0.5 to 1.2 millimeters thick. Between the cornea and the iris is a fluid that is mostly water called *aqueous humor* and the space this fluid occupies is the *anterior chamber.*

The cornea is composed of three main layers. The outer layer is called the *epithelium;* it has contact with the air and is bathed by tears during each blink. The epithelium is composed of several layers of epithelial cells. These cells can spread from one place to another to fill in gaps and can divide in several hours should it be necessary to produce more cells. New cells are formed at the inner layer, and as they age gradually work their way to the surface where they are washed away by tears.

The middle layer is called the *stroma.* It is the thickest layer and is composed of collagen fibrils. There is also considerable water in the stroma.

The inner layer is called the *endothelium.* It is only one cell thick. The cells found here do not reproduce and differ from epithelial cells in this respect. Thus, if an endothelial cell is damaged, neighboring cells must enlarge to cover the gap. In order for the cornea to remain clear it is necessary for the endothelium to be functioning properly. Otherwise, the cornea swells up with water from the aqueous humor and is not clear. A person with this problem would notice blurred vision.

Corneal Abrasion and Scar

The epithelium can get scratched by a fingernail, contact lens, tree branch, mascara application brush, or even by dust particles being blown in the air. Such a scratch is called a *corneal abrasion.* A corneal abrasion is extremely painful because the nerves that are normally covered by the epithelium are now exposed to the air. This extra stimulation also causes a muscle inside the eye to go into spasm, which adds to the pain. A patient with a corneal abrasion often describes a sharp, stabbing pain that may be worse when the lids move. There may be extreme sensitivity to light and excessive tearing. Some people, however, note only a mild sensation of something like an eyelash or piece of sand being in the eye. Generally, only a small area of the epithelium is scratched and other epithelial cells nearby can slide over the area to cover the defect and make the surface smooth again. It is imperative that the surface be smooth or else light will be distorted as it passes through the cornea.

To diagnose a corneal abrasion a small amount of fluorescein dye may be placed on the eye. A local anesthetic drop is used to relieve the pain and allow the examination to progress. The examiner then shines a blue light on the cornea and any scratched area then shows up. The rest of the eye is also examined, as previously described, to be sure that no other injury has occurred.

A drop is then placed on the eye to control the muscle spasm. An antibiotic ointment is applied and the lids are closed. A cotton patch is placed over the closed lids and taped into position. (The patch should be tight enough to prevent the lid from opening but not so tight as to be uncomfortable.) After the anesthetic drop wears off there will be some increase in pain but the eye should not be as painful as it was initially. The anesthetic drop cannot be used repeatedly because it loses its effect and also inhibits the healing process. Use of the anesthetic drop alone is dangerous because blinking is reduced and severe infections may occur that can result in total loss of vision. The patch prevents the blinking lids from washing away the newly forming cells and generally remains in place overnight. It may be necessary to use the patch longer. Healing usually occurs in a few days. If the patch should come off by accident, it is important to realize that the drop used to relax the muscle in spasm will also dilate the pupil and make it difficult to focus on close objects. The drop generally lasts two to four days. In some particularly difficult cases, as in a recurrent problem, a soft contact lens may be used as a bandage lens.

Sometimes the epithelial cells are only somewhat damaged and not actually abraded. This can occur after prolonged exposure to intense sunlight, such as lying on a beach all day or skiing on a very sunny day without proper sunglasses. Exposure to an arc-welding light without proper protection can also damage the epithelial cells. In this type of injury, the epithelial cells become swollen and do not function properly. There is about a 4- to 10-hour time lag from the time of injury to the time when the epithelial cells no longer function. This injury may be treated in the same manner described for a corneal abrasion. The following case is typical:

Case 23

Michael P. liked to go skiing and did so frequently. One day he forgot his sunglasses. He didn't buy new ones because the day was partly overcast and he didn't plan to ski long. Snow conditions were excellent, however, and he skied all day. That night he awoke about 2:00 A.M. with intense pain in his eyes. He called me, and upon examination I found that he had a corneal abrasion in each eye. He was treated with medication and patching and was back to normal a couple of days later. Even though the injury resolved without further complications, the pain that Michael initially had was an experience he would not like to repeat.

Overwearing contact lenses can also lead to epithelial damage and abrasion, as has been discussed. Fortunately, these types of epithelial injury generally heal quickly without any long-term damage to the cornea or to the eyesight. It is important to be properly evaluated, however, since complications, such as infection, can sometimes occur.

Problems can also occur in the stroma. For example, a traumatic injury may go deeper than the epithelial layer. The stroma heals by forming scar tissue. If the injury and resultant scar are off to one side of the cornea, there may be very little visual deficit. However, a scar in the center may cause some decrease in vision, depending on how large and how dense it is. The epithelial damage is treated as discussed before; the scar in the stroma will form over a period of days to weeks and may require a corneal transplant (see below).

The innermost layer of the cornea, the endothelium, can also have problems. As a person gets older it is normal for some of the endothelial cells to degenerate. The remaining endothelial cells enlarge to take their place. Sometimes there are not enough endothelial cells to cover the area, even though they can become quite large. When this happens the cornea swells up. This happens because the endothelial cells normally pump out excess water from the stroma and form a barrier to the water of the aqueous fluid in the anterior chamber. Vision becomes blurred when the cornea is swollen. Endothelial cells can also be damaged by trauma or during surgery on the eye. Again, a corneal transplant may be needed (see below).

Corneal Transplant

When there is a scar in the stroma that blocks vision or when there is swelling of the cornea from a problem with the endothelium, or another corneal problem, a corneal transplant may be performed. A corneal transplant involves replacing the central section (usually about a seven- to eight-millimeter diameter disc) of the patient's cornea with a section of the same size and shape from an individual who is deceased, the donor. Only human donor material is used. The donor cornea is checked to be sure it contains no scars and is generally taken from a younger individual so that there should be many well-functioning endothelial cells. However, corneas donated from older persons are frequently quite acceptable. Since only the cornea, which is clear, is transplanted, the color of the donor's eye does not matter. Nor, for that matter, does the donor's sex, race, or level of eyesight.

The cornea must be removed from the donor within a few hours after death and placed in a special solution to keep it fresh. It is generally used within a few days. There is a nationwide network of eye banks that arrange to transport and distribute donated corneas to individuals in need. Corneas from donors with certain eye problems, which cannot be used for transplant purposes, are used for research.

Only corneas that have been donated are used. Corneas are not bought and sold. Volunteer labor and charitable contributions are used to maintain the eye bank system. If you should wish to donate your corneas you should inform your family of your wishes and contact your local eye bank to be registered and obtain a donor identification card. Many states have a place on the driver's license to indicate whether one wishes to be a donor. Your ophthalmologist can answer further questions about this subject.

After the central part of the patient's cornea is removed, the previously prepared donor cornea is placed into position and sewn into place with microsurgical instruments. The actual surgery takes about one hour. See Chapter 7 for additional information on the surgical procedures.

In a successful surgery, the transplanted cornea remains clear. Rejection of the transplanted cornea is commonly a reason for an unsuccessful result. A variety of drops are used after the operation to keep the pupil at rest and to try to prevent infection and rejection of the donor cornea. The normal body tries to reject any foreign material whether it be a splinter of wood in the finger, a flu virus, or a transplanted tissue. Fortunately, most such rejection attempts can be controlled with medication. If the donated cornea is rejected, it becomes opaque and the patient notices decreased vision. A rejected cornea does not fall out of position. Another transplant can usually be performed if the patient wishes and it may be more successful.

After the swelling has resolved, it is frequently possible to improve vision further with the use of eyeglasses. The stitches may stay in place for one year or longer, although they are sometimes removed sooner, if they are causing a problem. Healing is slower than one might expect because every effort is made to keep blood vessels from growing into the wound in order to prevent a rejection episode; antibodies and certain cells in the blood are thought to cause the rejection response.

Corneal transplants are also performed for other diseases such as keratoconus and some metabolic diseases. Keratoconus means the cornea is shaped like a cone. Although the visual distortions caused by this abnormal shape can sometimes be helped with contact lenses and/or glasses, a corneal transplant is often needed. Certain metabolic diseases can cause corneal opacities for which a corneal transplant may also be helpful.

A corneal transplant can only help an individual with a problem with the cornea. A corneal transplant will not help a person who has retina problems or glaucoma. Usually when people refer to an "eye transplant" they are referring to a corneal transplant as described. Although some success with using sclera as a patch over weakened sclera has been noted, no other parts of the eye have been transplanted. Corneal transplants have a higher success rate when compared to other organ transplants so that if you do need to have one, you should approach the prospect with this in mind.

CATARACTS

A cataract simply means that the lens inside your eye is not clear. Light passes directly through a clear lens, but it is distorted when it passes through a lens that is not clear. When a cataract is more advanced, it means that the lens is less clear than in an early cataract. Sometimes you will hear people talk about a cataract "growing" or "ripening." These terms are somewhat misleading, because a cataract that is progressing is *not* like a cancer or tumor that grows and spreads. Also, it is not contagious. A better analogy is that of comparing a clear window with a frosted one. Early in life the lens is clear; gradually it becomes more opaque, like frosted glass.

The symptoms of a cataract are basically variations of blurred vision. Words such as cloudy, blurry, foggy, smoky, or the sensation that a film is over the eye or one's glasses or contact lenses are dirty are commonly used descriptions. The observation that lights are not bright enough is common, although vision may be better at night. Car headlights may create a dazzling effect and colored haloes may be seen around lights. It is important to realize that not everyone with a cataract uses these descriptions and also that there are other causes aside from a cataract for these symptoms, some more serious. A good eye examination can distinguish among these various causes.

Each one of us would develop a noticeable cataract if we lived long enough. Cataract development is basically part of the normal growth and development of the human body. The lens is a living tissue, derived from the same type of cells as skin except that the lens is organized "inside-out" compared to the skin. In the skin, new cells are made at the deeper levels and as they mature, they migrate to the outer area. The old cells on the outer levels are rubbed away by friction or washed away in a bath. In the case of the lens, the new cells are on the outside and the older cells lie toward the center. After a number of years the cells and cell debris in the center are packed so tightly that light does not go straight through the lens. Instead, there are opacities that bounce the light in different directions, much as a smudge would on clear window glass. Various terms such as immature, mature, and hypermature are used to describe various degrees of cataract development. This is the usual process of cataract formation. The rate of progression of a cataract in an individual person is variable. It may take a couple of years, from thc earliest sign of a cataract, for one person to develop a significant cataract and 20 or 30 years for another. The rate of progression between eyes in the same person can also vary considerably.

Since these cells are living and are part of the body, they are affected by diseases that can affect the whole body. For example, diabetes affects the amount of sugar in the blood and blood is distributed throughout your body. It is not uncommon for people with diabetes to develop cataracts somewhat earlier than others, because an abnormally changing blood sugar level causes abnormal swelling of the lens. This swelling can cause some of the cells in the lens to degenerate faster, so that opacities formed from this debris may appear somewhat sooner than in a normal individual.

A traumatic injury can damage lens cells and also lead to earlier cataract development. Babies can be born with a preexisting cataract if the lens cells are damaged during fetal development, as by rubella (measles) virus. Many other factors are known or suspected to be involved in cataract formation. Poor nutrition, exposure of the eyes to certain types of radiation, chronic inflammation, and various drugs are a few of these factors. In addition, some people seem to have an inherited tendency for significant cataracts at a somewhat earlier age than usual. Excessive use of the eyes does not appear to be a factor. Other than maintaining good general health, as outlined earlier, and avoiding trauma and the other precipitating causes listed, there does not appear to be any specific way to prevent cataract formation.

In some circumstances the opacities may be reduced. For example, when diabetes is out of control and opacities start to form, they may regress somewhat if the diabetes is brought back into control. If the opacities are toward the edge of the lens and not in the center they may not cause as much of a problem. If the opacities are located more toward the center of the lens, dilating the pupil may be somewhat helpful in reducing the symptoms. This technique is usually helpful for only a short time because the cataract progresses, but for some people it is of help. This is the type of eye drop people may be referring to if they say drops "decreased" their cataracts. The drops are really not decreasing the cataract, just allowing some light to go around the opacity. Sunglasses may be needed if dilation is used, and in fact, some people find sunglasses helpful anyway in reducing the symptoms. For other people, sunglasses make the symptoms more noticeable and they don't like to wear them. Glare from car headlights is a common problem, again depending on the location of the opacities.

Sometimes during cataract formation, the lens may change its power, for example, because of a small amount of swelling. If this is the case, changing eyeglasses may somewhat improve vision. It may improve vision enough to enable the individual to defer the operation for a year or more. Depending on the original prescription and the type of power change caused by the cataract, there may be a stage when one sees best without any glasses. More often, however, changing glasses will not improve vision, just as a magnifying glass doesn't help one see through frosted glass better.

There really is no way to remove the opacities without surgically removing the whole lens. This operation takes about one hour and is done in an operating room, frequently with a local anesthetic only. It has one of the highest success rates of any surgical procedure in medicine. Different surgical methods are discussed later.

When to Operate

When the individual is no longer able to do the things he or she wants to do and would be able to do if his or her vision were better, it is time to consider having the operation. For some people who are younger and quite active this time might be when the cataract is less advanced. An example might be an accountant who is supporting a family and needs to read small numbers. A somewhat older person who doesn't drive a car may be able to wait longer. A person who still has very good vision in one eye, even with a cataract in the other eye, may not need the operation until the vision in the better eye starts to diminish.

Generally the eye with the least vision is operated on first. Only under very special circumstances would both eyes ever be operated on at the same time, to avoid any complications that may affect both eyes. Many people, in fact, will choose never to have the second eye operated on if the result of the operation on the first eye is successful. Other people prefer the additional field of vision and increased depth perception and thus choose to have the second eye operated on after waiting a reasonable time between operations. Except for relatively rare circumstances, such as leaking of fluid from inside the lens, it is acceptable to defer a cataract operation. Your ophthalmologist can discuss these options with you in more detail.

There are other problems to be considered. The nerves in the back of the eye may not be working as well as they once did and if this is the case, removing the lens with opacities in it will not improve vision as much as one might have liked. An analogy would be finding out that cleaning a camera lens does not help the picture if the film is no good. In other words, there can be more than one reason why your vision has decreased.

Replacement Lenses

With cataracts, a replacement lens for the lens that is removed is needed. There are basically three ways to do this, each with advantages and disadvantages. First is the use of eyeglasses. Since all of the power of the lens must be replaced, these glasses are generally thicker than glasses people might wear before a cataract operation. The main advantages are that they are simple to put on and take off and have the lowest potential for further direct complications to the eye. The disadvantage is that unless the individual looks through the center or near the center of the glasses there will be some distortions, such as greater magnification, less peripheral vision, and more spherical aberration. This last effect causes doorways, for example, to appear as though they are bowed in, as one walks toward and through them. These distortions can cause one initially to misjudge distances, since objects appear to be located differently in space, and to have problems from not seeing objects off to the side. Methods of grinding the lenses for these glasses to reduce (but not eliminate) these distortions were discussed in Chapter 2. People can adapt to these distortions but it does take more time and practice to do so than with glasses one may have worn when younger. Bifocals are prescribed to enable one to read. These glasses are sometimes called *aphakic glasses,* since a person who does not have his original lens inside his eye is termed *aphakic.* (A person with his original lens is termed *phakic*).

The second way to replace the lost lens power is to use a contact lens, either the hard or soft type. This method has the advantage of greatly reducing the distortions caused by cataract glasses. This is so because the lens is closer to its normal position. One disadvantage is that the individual must be able to put the contact lens on the eye every morning and take it off every night, or have someone who can do it for him. Many older people can learn to do this, but some people with arthritis or a tremor cannot do it easily. Contact lenses can cause corneal abrasions, although these generally heal fairly rapidly. Continuous wear or extended wear lenses are now being used for some aphakic individuals. However, these lenses are more fragile than hard lenses or regular soft lenses, since they have a higher water content. They frequently tear and need to be replaced as often as every few months. Reading glasses are still generally needed with the use of any contact lens.

The third method of lens replacement is to insert a plastic lens inside the eye at the time of the original operation, an *intraocular lens* or *implant.* This method has been used in the last 10 years or so. It has the advantage of being closest to the original position of the lens so there are much fewer distortions, and it stays in permanently. For a person who is not able to wear a contact lens and who has severe problems with cataract glasses, an intraocular lens would be helpful. The disadvantage is that any complication that occurs is potentially much more serious and can result in total loss of vision. These complications are slightly more frequent than with the other methods but are still fairly rare. Complications might include a greater risk of infection, bleeding, high pressure inside the eye (glaucoma), and problems with the cornea that may even require a corneal transplant. There are certain cases of chronic inflammation when an intraocular lens cannot be used. The intraocular lens causes a certain amount of inflammation by itself and various drugs (usually given as drops or ointments) are used to control this problem. However, if inflammation is already a problem, it may be quite difficult to control with the added inflammation from the intraocular lens and so it would generally not be used in such a case. Certain corneal problems, an unsuccessful result on the first eye, and other reasons may also be contraindications to the use of an intraocular lens. In addition, most people, even with successful intraocular lenses, still need reading glasses and sometimes distance glasses to see clearly. These glasses, however, generally are not as thick as the cataract glasses mentioned previously and do not have the same distortions.

There are many types of intraocular lenses. The technology in this field is rapidly changing. Some lenses are placed in front of the iris, some overlap the iris, and still others are placed completely behind the iris (see Fig. 18). The shape as well as the material of the lens and of the loops varies. The appropriate power is determined by using the prescription for the current glasses; sometimes the curvature of the cornea is measured with a keratometer and the length of the eye is measured by using a technique called ultrasound. Your

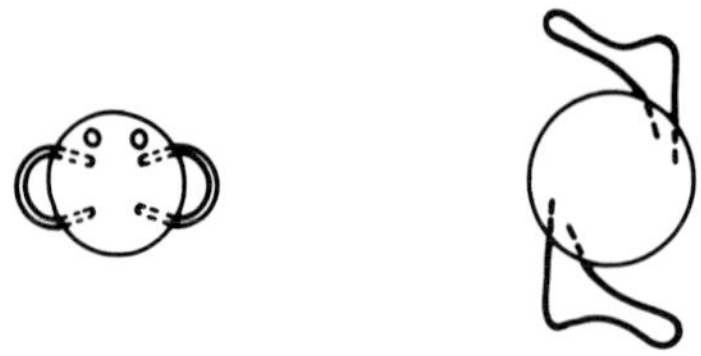

FIGURE 18. Intraocular lens. Some examples of the wide variety of styles and designs of intraocular lenses.

ophthalmologist will decide which type of lens is best for you should you decide to have an intraocular lens inserted.

People who see well in one eye and have a cataract in the other eye may decide not to have surgery at all. Deferring the operation, except as mentioned earlier, does *not* harm either eye. The operation can always be done should the vision in the better eye decrease. However, if such a person decides to have the operation when the vision in the the other eye is still quite good, because he or she requires better depth perception, for example, the choices for a replacement lens are more limited. If the first option is chosen, that is, eyeglasses, they cannot use both eyes together because the images are magnified differently, giving the sensation of double vision. In order to use both eyes together, either a contact lens or an intraocular lens must be used. The contact lens is close enough to the original lens position to reduce the magnification difference to a level that generally does not cause double vision. Many people find the use of the contact lens an inconvenience that is not needed as long as they see well out of one eye, and they often stop using the contact lens. It does not hurt the eye, however, to discontinue using the contact lens for this reason. The intraocular lens runs the risk of the complications previously discussed and some people think it is not worth this risk if one eye sees well. Other people think just the opposite, that is, that this is a reason that makes the risk more tolerable. The following cases describe several people's experiences with the same visual problem:

Case 24

Ethel R. was an 86-year-old woman who had ten grandchildren and three great-grandchildren. She had been quite active earlier in her life but now lived a less hectic life in her apartment. She enjoyed visits from her various children and grandchildren and wrote letters to those who lived in other cities. When they came to visit, she was still able to host the family dinner.

Ethel's vision had always been quite good. However, recently she noticed that everything was dimmer than before and that she needed additional light to read. Her children were concerned and brought her to see me.

Cataracts were the cause of her difficulties and we discussed the various possibilities. She decided that since she was still able to read a large-print newspaper and write letters to her friends and relatives that she would defer surgery for now. She had had a bad experience in the hospital the year before and did not now want to risk repeating that experience. She realized that she could have surgery later if her vision became more of a handicap. Her family and I concurred with her decision.

Case 25

John S. was a 50-year-old accountant who truly enjoyed his work. He liked to be involved in actually adding and subtracting the small figures in the various columns, even though he had assistants to do most of that sort of bookkeeping. He began noticing difficulty in doing this fine work and came to see me.

At first both he and I thought he just needed a change in his bifocals. This would be expected in a person his age and he had been told to expect this when he first began wearing them. A refraction, however, showed that changing his glasses did not help. Further examination revealed moderately dense cataracts, more dense in one eye than the other. When I told him that the cataracts were causing most of his problem, he said that he had been afraid of that since both his mother and grandmother had had moderately dense cataracts at the age of 50.

We discussed the various possibilities and John decided to have surgery with a contact lens to be used as a replacement lens. He thought he should be able to learn to wear contacts since his children were happy with them. An intraocular lens was not chosen since John thought of himself as young with many more years to live. He expected further refinements in technique and thought he could have surgery on the second eye some years later if the contact lens was unsatisfactory. I agreed with John's decision.

Case 26

Charles S. was a 68-year-old man with a moderately dense cataract in one eye. In addition, he had arthritis in his fingers, which made it difficult to perform fine manipulations. He was otherwise quite alert and active. He chose to have surgery with insertion of an intraocular lens, which was successfully completed.

Surgical Techniques

Your ophthalmologist will select the surgical technique that he or she thinks is most appropriate in your case should you develop cataracts. Some people, however, are interested in knowing more about these techniques and so they are discussed in this section.

There is a variety of different surgical techniques that can be used to remove the lens from the eye. One method is called an *intracapsular cataract extraction* and involves several steps. After an incision has been made, an enzyme solution may be injected to dissolve the zonules that hold the lens in position. Sometimes this is not necessary in older individuals. An instrument called a *cryoprobe* is placed under the cornea and on the lens and is "frozen" to the lens. The cryoprobe and lens are then carefully withdrawn from the eye. This method has the advantage of removing the complete lens and the thin capsule surrounding the lens. If the capsule is not removed it often becomes opacified and it may be necessary to cut an opening in it at a later time. This last procedure is not as complex as the original operation and may take only a few minutes, but it does involve another surgical procedure with some risk. The lens itself, however, once removed, does not grow back. Sometimes this opacification of the capsule causes patients to think their cataract has grown back. When the entire capsule is not removed, it is called an *extracapsular cataract extraction.* The advantage of not removing the capsule is that certain types of intraocular lenses are designed for use with the back capsule still in place. It is also thought that there may be somewhat less swelling and fewer retinal problems if this technique is employed.

An extracapsular type of cataract extraction is performed in children because at this age the back capsule of the lens is firmly attached to the vitreous, which is firmly attached to the retina, which contains the nerves. An attempt to remove this capsule may, therefore, cause damage to the nerves. In older adults this is generally not a problem.

Phacoemulsification is a type of extracapsular cataract extraction. This technique involves inserting an instrument into the eye that is about the diameter of a pen. This instrument shatters the lens into small parts by ultrasonic vibration. These small pieces can then be sucked out of the eye through an opening in the instrument. Irrigation is used to help remove the pieces. This is not the same as a laser. A laser is not used to remove a cataract. The advantage of phacoemulsification is that the incision is not as large as in the other techniques, since the whole lens is not pulled through intact. The human lens is about the size of an aspirin tablet. Thus, there are fewer stitches. If, however, an intraocular lens is also to be inserted, the incision must be opened a little to allow the intraocular lens to fit through. This incision, however, is still not as large as the ones for the other procedures. The advantage of a smaller incision is that there is less chance of infection, fewer distortions from changing the shape of the cornea, less possibility of wound breakdown, and somewhat faster recovery. It is possible, however, to damage the back side of the cornea (endothelium) with the probe, and the capsule does remain in place, so this technique also has disadvantages.

At the time of any of these operations, a small cut is made in the iris or a small piece of iris is removed. This cut is often not visible since the upper lid covers it. It is called a *peripheral iridotomy* or *peripheral iridectomy* and is done to create a permanent access to the drainage channel for the aqueous fluid. Once the lens is removed, the normal anatomy has been changed and this extra opening can prevent certain complications, such as one type of glaucoma, from occurring.

All of these procedures are generally performed with the surgeon using a magnification device, usually an operating microscope. The newer sutures are quite thin, in fact, finer than a human hair. Some are difficult to see without magnification. Needles are shaped for ease of use and are quite sharp. These advances, along with the various antibiotic, anti-inflammatory, anesthetic, and enzymatic drugs used, are the reasons why cataract surgery is now so successful.

Postoperative Information

It is important to realize that there is a rehabilitation period for the eye no matter which technique is used to remove the lens and no matter which type of replacement lens is employed. Later in the day, after the operation has been performed, most patients are encouraged to get out of bed with assistance and to sit in a chair or walk with help. Depending on the vision in the other eye, temporary cataract glasses may be prescribed at the time of discharge from the hospital. The final prescription for cataract glasses is generally not given until at least six weeks after the operation and frequently longer (three months or more). This time period is necessary for the wound to heal and for the swelling to subside. In addition, sutures may need to be removed before a final prescription is given. An intraocular lens will enable one to have better vision at the time of discharge from the hospital, but for the best vision that one will eventually have, these patients usually also need to wait several weeks. It should be realized, however, that even without glasses, a contact lens, or an intraocular lens, an aphakic patient still has some vision. For example, he can recognize large objects and perhaps even some people's faces.

Your ophthalmologist will instruct you in what sort of care needs to be given to your eye and what sort of activities are permitted. Usually only the eye that was operated on has a patch. The other eye can still be used during the rehabilitation period. A number of visits to your ophthalmologist's office will be needed to ensure that your postoperative recovery is progressing normally.

One of the problems that your doctor will look out for is a retinal detachment. This is discussed further in Chapter 5. It is important to realize that about two percent of the people who have cataract surgery will have a retinal detachment, and it needs to be repaired within a few days for the best results. Until you have your final lens correction, it is hard for you to tell if you have such a detachment. During this period, however, you will be seen frequently enough to have your ophthalmologist diagnose it. Later, though, you will need to be aware of the symptoms so that you can seek prompt attention should you have one. Such a retinal detachment may even occur several years after the initial cataract operation. The symptoms include the sensation of a curtain coming down over your field of vision or coming up into your field of vision, or a shadow off to the side. In addition, lightning flashes or sparkling lights may be noticed. If you clean your glasses or contact lens and the shadow does not go away, you should call your ophthalmologist so you can be seen the same day or next day. If you are out of town, you should consult a local ophthalmologist rather than wait several days or weeks until you come home.

As a last comment, remember that deferring cataract surgery, except in rare and special circumstances, does not affect the technical difficulty of performing the operation. If these special circumstances are applicable in your case, your ophthalmologist will tell you so and discuss why in more detail. This operation can be performed successfully on people who are over 90 years old and in people who have many other medical problems.

GLAUCOMA

Glaucoma is a condition where the pressure inside the eye is too high. The aqueous humor fluid is mostly water and fills up the anterior chamber, which is the space between the front of the iris and the back of the cornea. The aqueous humor supplies nutrients to the eye and removes waste products. It is produced by a group of glands in the *ciliary body.* The fluid enters the eye from the glands at a certain rate and must also exit at the same rate to keep the pressure the same and in a normal range. If excess fluid is produced or if the fluid cannot drain quickly enough, pressure builds up. If the pressure is high enough for a long enough time, damage can occur to the nerves in the eye. This condition is called *glaucoma.* Problems can also occur if the fluid is not produced fast enough or drains out too fast. The pressure then decreases too much and the eye becomes too soft to function normally. This condition is different from glaucoma.

A common problem in older people is that the drainage channels are not as wide as they used to be. Various deposits and other debris tend to clog them. In infants or young children, the drainage channels may not have been wide enough originally. In all of these cases the pressure inside the eye can build up to unacceptable levels.

The nerves that are affected first are the ones that enable a person to see things on the side of the field of vision while concentrating on looking at an object straight ahead, the *peripheral vision.* The vision used to read or to see clear detail, the *central vision,* is affected last. Damage in the early stages is often not noticed by a person for this reason, and in order to detect early changes, a general eye examination is needed periodically. The late stage of nearly complete loss of peripheral vision gives one the sensation of looking through a narrow tube. Ultimately, if glaucoma is untreated, loss of both the peripheral and central vision can occur. It should be noted that there are other causes aside from glaucoma for loss of peripheral vision.

There are four main tests that are used to check for glaucoma. In a general eye examination the pressure inside the eye is measured and the nerves inside the eye are directly observed. The pressure is called the *intraocular pressure.* It is not the same as blood pressure. A better view of the nerves is obtained through a dilated pupil and so frequently it is necessary to dilate the eyes for this examination. If both of these tests are normal, nothing further is generally done other than routine follow-up examinations.

If either one is abnormal, a contact lens is placed on the eye through use of a local anesthetic drop to enable observation of the fluid drainage sites. This contact lens has a mirror placed at an angle that allows the observer to see the drainage channels. The technique is called *gonioscopy.* A different part of this lens enables the observer to have a magnified stereoscopic view of the optic nerve head, which is a somewhat different view than other techniques permit. Photographs of the optic nerve head are sometimes taken to allow better comparison of changes that may be observed in subsequent examinations. This is not always needed, however, in order to be able to make such comparisons.

Testing of the visual field is also done. This study takes about one hour and does not hurt. While the patient looks straight ahead, lights of different sizes and degree of brightness are flashed to different sides, one at a time. Each time a light is seen, the patient pushes a buzzer to inform the examiner that a light has been seen. These responses are recorded on a graph and measure how the nerves are actually working in a wide field, hence the name (visual field), of the test. Since the patient is looking straight ahead while the lights are flashed to the side, the peripheral vision is measured. The nerves may be working fine even if they don't look as normal as they should, or even if the pressure is at the upper end of the normal range or even slightly beyond. Visual fields are discussed further at the end of this chapter.

If any of these studies is abnormal, treatment may be needed. Sometimes, repeating some of these tests a few months later is initially recommended, and such a patient is called a "glaucoma suspect" rather than an individual with glaucoma. In addition, drops or pills may be prescribed that act either to reduce the rate at which fluid enters the eye or to speed up the rate at which it leaves. A continuous release form of one type of drop, called an Ocusert®, is available. The small packet containing the drug is wafer-thin and is placed under the upper lid. It is changed about once a week. This method of drug delivery is more expensive than drops, but some people find it more convenient. Surgery is sometimes needed to enlarge the drainage sites, but this is generally only used after medication has failed to keep the pressure within an acceptable range or when there is evidence of progressive nerve damage. For most people, the problem is controlled relatively easily by the use of medication and these people often do not notice any visual deficit.

There are a number of other studies that can be done to further clarify the problem. They are not performed as universally and include such techniques as tonography and various provocative tests. Another technique involves measuring the intraocular pressure at different times during the day or even night to plot what is called a diurnal curve. This technique can show if there is one particular time of day when the pressure is highest. If such additional studies are needed, your ophthalmologist can explain them to you in more detail.

A number of organizations sponsor glaucoma screening programs. It should be realized that only the intraocular pressure at one particular time is measured at these sessions. The nerves, drainage sites, and fields are not measured or observed and thus there could still be a problem even if the pressure is found to be normal during the one isolated measurement. It should also be realized that even if this one pressure measurement is abnormal that it does not necessarily mean that glaucoma is present. These screening sessions are not a substitute for a complete eye examination. They are simply rough screening measurements and have value only if the results are interpreted and used properly.

One of the main problems in treatment of glaucoma lies in convincing the patient that he needs to use eye drops or other medication, generally every day or several times a day (usually for the rest of his life), when he or she can still see well and has no pain in the eye. After a period of time many people become lax in using their drops or pills and damage can then occur. Some people are bothered by various side effects of some of the medications. All drugs, unfortunately, have some sort of undesirable side effects that are particularly bothersome in some individuals. Frequently, however, alternative equally effective medications are available that may make treatment more tolerable. You should discuss any problems of this sort that you may be having with your doctor to see if a solution can be found to the problem. It is preferable to discuss the problem rather than to stop using the medicine and pretend that you really are using it. Once damage has occurred, nothing can reverse it. The medicines keep the damage from getting worse. They do not repair damage that has already occurred. It is most important that these ideas be understood. If you have any questions, be sure to ask them. The following case illustrates what can happen when you don't:

Case 27

Joan N. was told that the pressure inside her eye was slightly high and that it should be rechecked. She moved to another city. She did finally have the pressure rechecked and it was too high at this time as well. A visual field examination showed early damage to her nerves resulting in a small loss of field. She was given a diagnosis of chronic open-angle glaucoma, the most common type, and was placed on medication. Joan did not like using the drops and when she ran out she did not get more for this reason and because she was getting ready to be married. She moved to another city after the wedding and did not do anything further about her eyes until she applied for a job and was required to have an eye examination.

She arranged an appointment and the intraocular pressure was again found to be too high. She was to have her old records transferred but she could not get them since in the several years since she was first told she had a problem, the other doctor had retired and the records could not be located. She missed several appointments and finally had another field study. This time severe loss of field was noted in one eye and moderate loss in the other. The loss was so severe that she almost did not get the job for which she was applying.

This news jolted her and now she is quite careful to use all her medications and keep all her appointments. She always has an extra supply of medication and has a copy of the prescription in her purse and at home. She is hopeful that no further deterioration will occur since she knows that the damage that has already occurred is not reversible.

The most common form of glaucoma is the type discussed in Case 27, that is, *chronic open-angle glaucoma.* It slowly progresses and you probably would not be aware of it unless you were noted to have it during a general eye examination or if it were very far advanced. This is why glaucoma has been described as a "thief in the night" who silently steals your vision without your being aware of it until it is too late. This form of glaucoma is usually not seen in people under the age of 35 and it may run in families. Thus, if your parents had glaucoma, you should be checked for it. Medication can generally control the disease by keeping the pressure low enough to prevent further damage.

Another type of glaucoma, called *acute narrow-angle glaucoma,* is much less common than the chronic open-angle type discussed above. Acute glaucoma occurs suddenly and a person with this problem may notice intense eye pain, headache, nausea, vomiting, and blurred vision. It is important to treat this problem immediately. This disease occurs when the drainage channels for the aqueous humor are suddenly blocked. The pressure inside the eye then rapidly rises to an unacceptable level and various medications must be used to reduce the pressure as soon as possible. This is not the sort of problem that you can treat yourself. Generally, after the initial attack a surgical procedure, called a peripheral iridectomy, is performed to try to prevent a recurrence. This procedure creates a permanent alternate route for the fluid to gain access to the drainage channels.

Still another type of glaucoma is one caused by or related to another problem, so-called *secondary glaucoma.* For example, an injury may disrupt the arrangement of the drainage channels and they may no longer function normally. Secondary glaucoma can also occur after surgical procedures and in chronic inflammatory conditions. In certain diseases, such as diabetes mellitus, new blood vessels can grow into the drainage channels and this can also lead to bleeding with resultant scarring and occlusion of the channels. Protein leakage from a hypermature cataract, although rarely seen in the United States, is another such cause. Treatment depends on the cause but usually includes medication of the sort discussed for chronic glaucoma.

Congenital glaucoma means you were born with glaucoma. It is rare and is seen in infants. The eyes may appear large and there may be an unusual amount of tearing and excessive sensitivity to light. An ophthalmologic examination can determine if an infant has this problem. It is caused by improper formation of the drainage channels. Treatment includes surgical enlargement of the drainage sites.

New Developments

For types of glaucoma that do not respond favorably to medication or the usual surgical procedures, a new procedure is currently being evaluated. It involves the insertion of an artificial valve at the site of the drainage channels. This procedure is experimental and is done in only a few places; it is not yet clear whether it will be a useful additional technique.

Other new advances in the treatment of glaucoma include the introduction of newer drugs that are more effective in controlling intraocular pressure. Some of the newer drugs also have less troublesome side effects. Other new drugs do not need to be used as frequently as some of the older ones. New methods of delivering the drugs are also being developed, as mentioned earlier. In some cases, a laser is used to make a peripheral iridectomy and experiments are currently being performed to test the usefulness of a laser in treating chronic open-angle glaucoma. Your ophthalmologist can discuss with you whether any of these developments would be appropriate in your case.

Visual Fields

The visual field examination has been discussed in relation to glaucoma. Visual fields are also evaluated for a variety of other prob-

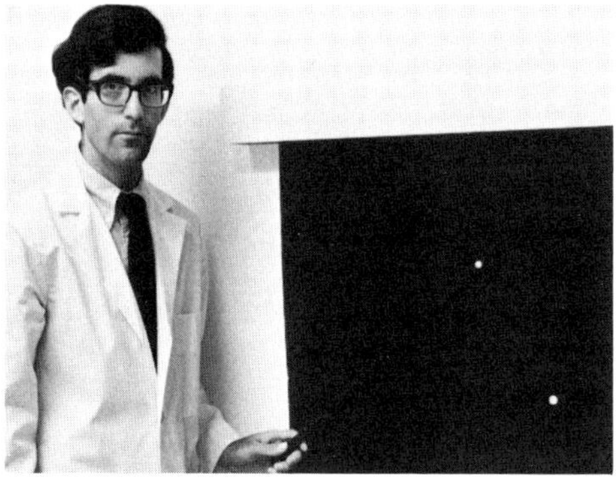

FIGURE 19. Tangent screen. This is one technique for measuring visual fields. The targets are variable in size and are placed in different areas of the visual field.

lems, such as endocrine and neurologic diseases. This section discusses the test in more detail.

There are three main ways to measure peripheral visual fields. The least accurate but the quickest is called the confrontation technique. It is used as a rough screening technique. The examiner and the patient look at each other and the examiner's fingers are brought from the periphery in toward the central line of vision. The patient signals when he can see the fingers. This method may be used to detect large defects and a variation of it can be used to test infants or small children.

The tangent screen is more accurate but is basically the same idea (see Fig. 19). The patient looks at a target on the screen and smaller objects are introduced into the field. The patient again signals when he sees the object.

The Goldmann perimeter or its various similar models is the most sensitive way to detect visual field defects, such as those caused by early glaucoma or certain other diseases. Again, the patient looks at a central target with his chin in a chin rest and this time lights are flashed in various locations inside a hemispheric dome that partially surrounds the patient's head. The size and intensity of the lights can be varied by the examiner. The examiner can also tell if the patient moves his eye from the fixation target. A graph is prepared by an ingenious system of interlocking arms that correlate the position of the flashed light to the proper place on the graph paper. This method is the most sensitive because the lights can be made quite

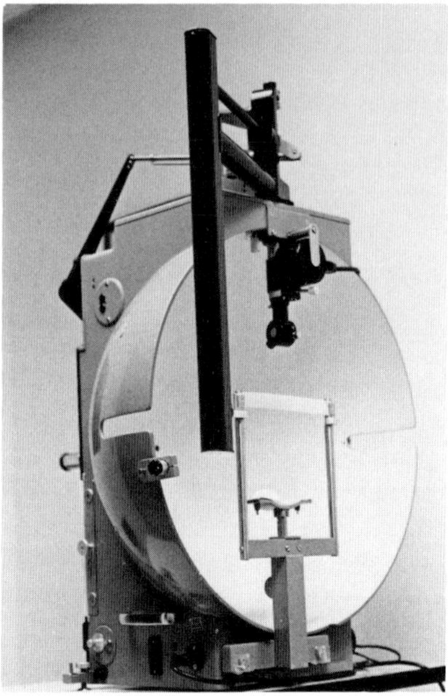

FIGURE 20. Goldmann perimeter, front. This is the instrument generally used to measure the visual fields for glaucoma. This view shows where the patient would sit. Lights are flashed from a moveable arm onto the hemisperic screen.

small and the precise correlation of the graph to the place where the light is flashed allows one to check for reproducibility of response in very small areas. Thus, very early signs of damage to the nerves can be detected. This method is used to diagnose and follow glaucoma and other diseases.

In all three methods each eye is tested separately. A patch is used to cover the other eye.

What these tests are measuring is the sensitivity of nerve cells in various locations to the target. There are approximately 1 million of these nerves in each eye. They are distributed mostly in the back hemisphere of the eye; each responds if stimulated from the appropriate direction. Thus, the visual field test measures whether a group of nerves in the area stimulated will respond properly, that is, whether the patient sees the object. If, for example, a light is flashed in a particular area but the patient does not see it, one can say that there is a visual field defect and that the nerves in that area or their

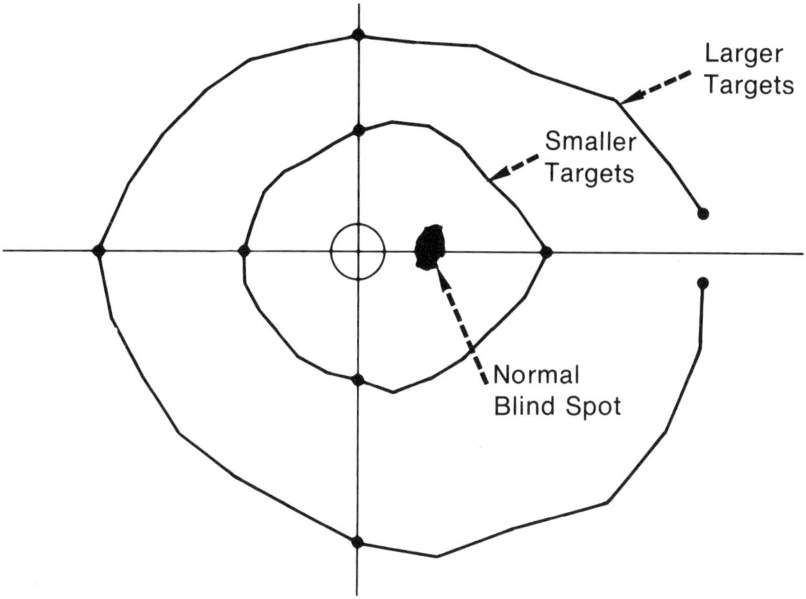

FIGURE 21. Visual fields, normal. This is a typical normal visual field study. The larger, brighter targets are seen farther on the periphery. The normal blind spot is marked.

connections are not functioning properly. These visual field defects are usually so small, at least in the early stages, that a person does not notice them by himself. It is only when they are actively tested for that they become evident.

In glaucoma, it is important to detect the earliest sign of damage since treatment can then be started, hopefully to prevent further damage that would become noticeable by a patient. The visual field examination is repeated from time to time to see if a defect noted on a previous examination is the same or if it has enlarged, or if a new defect has appeared. Treatment may be changed if new or changing defects are noted. In some people the field examination is normal, even though there may be other signs suggestive of glaucoma. In this case the field examination is usually repeated at another time. A

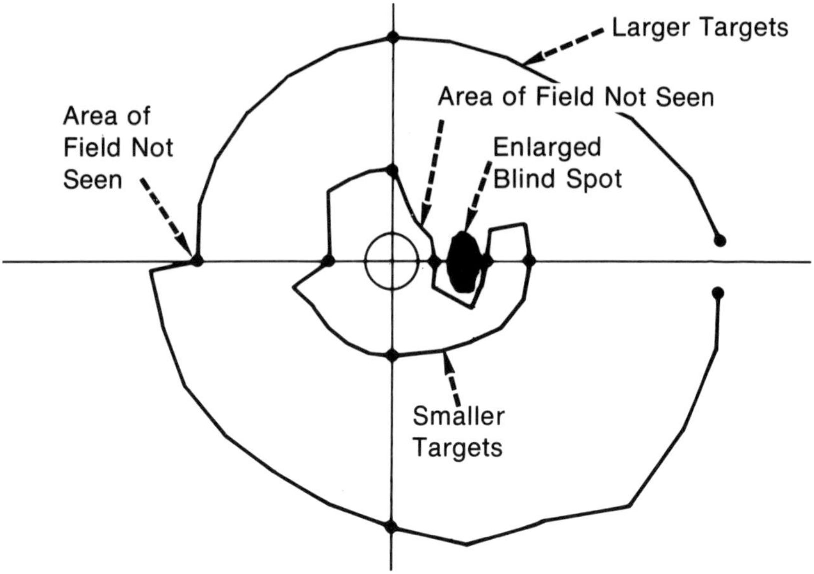

FIGURE 22. Visual fields, abnormal. This is an abnormal visual field study, such as might be seen in a case of glaucoma. One can see the area where the targets are not seen.

patient is generally not said to have glaucoma unless there is a field defect that is consistent and reproducible.

A normal visual field is approximately round to oval. Irregularities in the pattern suggest that nerves in that area are not functioning properly. The diameter of the field is related to the size and intensity of the test objects. If a large area of nerves is severely affected, the patient may notice that there is a section of the field of vision that is not seen. For example, if the entire right side of the field was missing in a given patient, such a patient would not be able to perceive his hand moving in that field unless he turned his head or eyes. Examples of normal and abnormal fields are shown.

There is one visual field defect that is normal, and it is called the physiologic blind spot. It occurs where the 1 million nerves of the retina are gathered into one bundle called the optic nerve. The optic

FIGURE 23. Normal Blind Spot. The normal blind spot occurs because there are no photoreceptors in the area where the optic nerve leaves the eye. It can be demonstrated by holding this book about 15 inches away and looking at the left mark with the left eye closed. Slowly bring the book closer while continuing to look at the left mark. Note that the right mark vanishes when the book is about 10 inches away. This is the physiologic blind spot. Bring the book even closer and it will reappear when it is again focused on an area of the retina where there are photoreceptors.

nerve leaves the eyeball and connects to other nerves in the brain. This area of the eye does not have photoreceptors, so one does not perceive an object that has an image focused in this area. The normal blind spot is rather small, but it is possible to demonstrate it to oneself by closing the left eye and looking with the right eye at the left mark in the figure above (see instructions in legend).

As has been mentioned, visual field defects occur in many other diseases besides glaucoma. A few of these would be other problems with the retina, some tumors, and problems with blood vessels. Your ophthalmologist is trained to decide what the cause of a particular defect might be. Sometimes additional tests are needed.

Recently, automated machines have been introduced to measure the visual field. It is not clear if these machines will be as good or perhaps better than the current techniques employed. In any event, the interpretation of the examination is necessary for it to be useful.

It is also possible to measure the central field or, more accurately, the area just next to the central vision. The idea is basically the same. In one technique, called an Amsler grid, a grid of lines is held about 13 inches from the eye and the patient is instructed to look at a central target and point out any parts of the grid that seem to be absent. Central vision is discussed further in Chapter 5.

CHAPTER 5

Conditions of the Back of the Eye

DECREASED CENTRAL VISION AND LOW VISION AIDS

Everyone has two different visual systems in each eye. One system allows perception of fine detail and is called central vision. The other enables a person to see things to the side while concentrating on looking at an object straight ahead and is called peripheral vision. Many diseases that affect one system generally do not affect the other. (Peripheral vision was discussed in the previous chapter.)

Central vision is used to read or sew, for example. Problems with central vision cause difficulty in doing these things. Total loss of central vision does *not* mean one is blind; however, one criteria for *legal* blindness is loss of central vision. Again, this does not mean *total* blindness. Peripheral vision is adequate to find the way around a room, to recognize faces to a certain extent, and to see large objects, such as obstacles in a path. If a person has only peripheral vision, he or she can still lead an independent life.

A variety of organizations and aids of various sorts are available to help people with decreased vision maintain their independence. These are listed at the end of this section. Some of these organizations also help people who are totally blind, so the word blind may appear in their names. This does *not* mean that a person will end up totally blind if it is recommended that their services be used.

Causes

The main difficulty in the eye that causes decreased central vision is a problem with certain nerve cells located in the part of the retina directly in the back of the eye. This area is called the *macula* and contains between 50,000 and 100,000 nerves. The total number of nerves in one eye is about 1 million. This explains why vision can be decreased but not completely lost. If, for example, half of the nerves in the macula are not working as well as they should, central vision will be decreased. There are many reasons why the nerves in the macula may not be functioning normally. Causes include such things as scars, inflammations, infections, trauma, degeneration, problems with blood vessels in the area, and many others (see Figs. 24, 25). Depending on the cause both eyes may be affected. However, even if both eyes become affected many years may pass before the second eye has significantly reduced vision. Many of the various optical aids try to make better use of the remaining functional nerves.

One way to do this is to have a larger image so that more nerves are exposed to the object of regard. This is why magnification of various kinds is used. The problem is that the laws of optics cause a smaller area to be seen when the magnification is greater. It is not practical to magnify a word so much that only part of one letter is seen at a time.

Learning to Cope

In order to get useful magnification for reading, for example, a variety of techniques are available. Magnifying lenses can be worn as spectacles, held in the hand, or placed in a rigid stand that rests on the page. (The stand magnifiers are more stable if a patient has a tremor.) Sometimes vision is better if one looks slightly to the side of the object he or she wants to see. Larger print books and magazines are available in a surprisingly large number and variety of topics. Closed circuit television can be used to project print onto a larger television-type screen.

Telescopes can be used for magnification of an object far away,

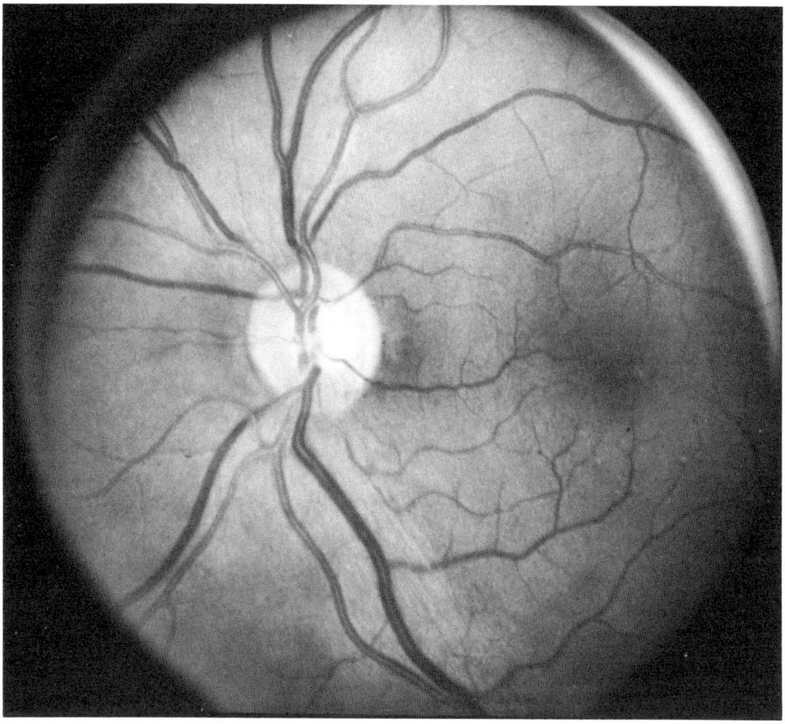

FIGURE 24. Normal fundus. This is a photograph of a typical normal fundus, as seen with the indirect ophthalmoscope. Note the arteries and veins, which are the major blood vessels. The optic disc is where the nerve fibers leave the eyeball and form the large bundle of nerves called the optic nerve. The macula is where the nerves that give central vision are located. When the eyes are focused on a given object, light waves go straight back to the macula. One can see that the macula is a small area compared to the whole retinal area.

for example, to read the number on a bus or a street sign. Frequently, a combination of devices and techniques produces an acceptable, even if not perfect, result. The following case shows how it may be possible to find a useful, although not ideal solution:

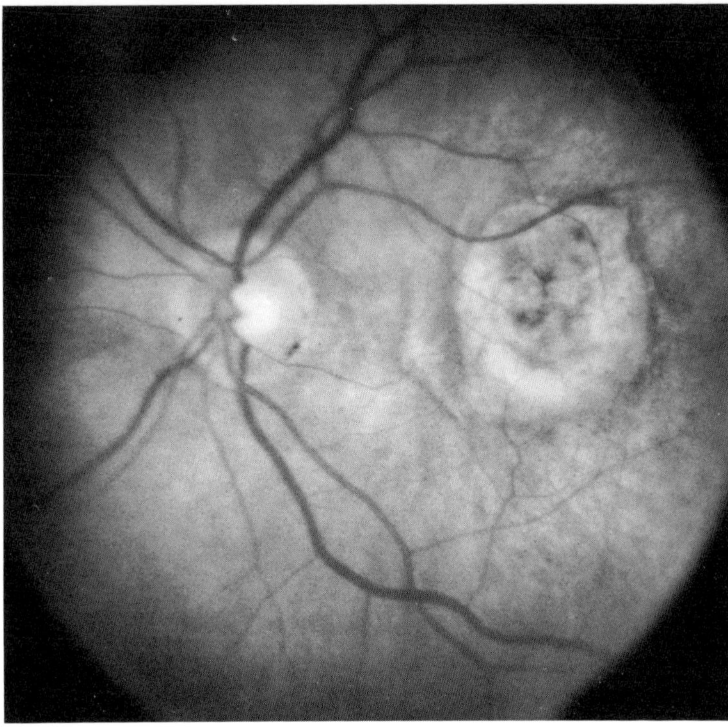

FIGURE 25. Abnormal fundus. In this example, one can see a large scar in the macula. This person would have difficulty reading since this task requires a functioning macula, but peripheral vision should be normal.

Case 28

Mark C. was a businessman who enjoyed his work. When he began noticing decreased vision, he became quite alarmed. He had problems reading the newspaper, and difficulty reading the number on the bus. He was noted to have macular degeneration as the cause of his problem and had been told that there was nothing that could be done. He came to me for another opinion.

While I agreed with the diagnosis I thought that it was worth trying to use various optical aids to help Mark retain his independence. He found it useful to use a dilating drop to allow more light to reach his retina and he used a telescope to read the bus numbers. He was able to use a stand magnifier to read the various papers he needed for his work. Thus, in his case, a combination of aids was helpful even though the actual condition could not be reversed.

Lighting is important and by varying the type, intensity, and direction to reduce glare, greater vision is obtained. Glare can also be reduced by covering parts of the page not being read with a nonreflective material. Many people find that a gooseneck type of lamp that can be easily adjusted is useful. Having the light coming over a shoulder onto the page is often helpful.

Line guides may be useful for reading and in writing. Visors may be of benefit in reducing glare outdoors. Sunglasses may also be helpful.

People find it useful to have a particular place in their homes where all of these aids are located so that conditions are constant and they are not always juggling different influences. For people for whom none of these techniques is of help, quite a large number and variety of recorded books are available free through public libraries. Some are available as records and others as cassette tapes. Record players and tape machines are also provided free of charge and are designed to be used easily by people with decreased or absent vision.

A number of other common objects that are used every day have been modified to make it possible and safer for a person with reduced central vision to employ them. They range from simple things like larger print playing cards and larger telephone numbering dials, to clocks with hands that can be touched and knives with safety devices and controls to regulate the size of a slice and to protect the fingers.

It is important to keep a positive attitude about a visual handicap. Realizing that certain emotional reactions are common may make it easier to deal with these feelings. For example, some people have a diminished sense of personal worth if they have decreased or absent vision. These people can be uncomfortable meeting new people and even interacting with friends. A feeling of loss of independence if one is no longer able to drive can be discouraging to some people. Many people have anxieties about hurting themselves from a fall or from bumping into something. Most people find it hard to verbalize these various fears and feelings, but one's doctor should be consulted if these feelings are being experienced.

As an example of how much it is possible to do, even with little or no vision, one should be aware that in several major ski resorts in Colorado there are programs for blind skiers. These individuals can ski on slopes of intermediate difficulty with an instructor who helps keep other skiers from coming too close and who is present in case of certain problems. These blind individuals are able to ski without holding onto someone and without having a rope attached. In fact, the techniques used in the program have actually been shown to be of value in helping to teach people with normal vision to ski. Instruction for normal individuals now includes certain maneuvers that are performed with the eyes closed, which can help a person to develop a better sense of balance.

The main things to keep in mind regarding a central vision problem are:

1. In most cases one should retain peripheral vision, since the most common cause of this process affects only central vision. Of course, one can still get any other problem that anyone else gets but it is unlikely that there will be two major problems in one person.
2. Various aids are available and should be used for whatever help they can provide. It is *not* an embarrassment or admission of inadequacy to try them.
3. Central vision, if lost, does not return. There is no magic cure. The best thing to do is to try to make the most of what one still has.

Sources of Help and Information for People with Decreased Central Vision

Optical Aids. Samples of various types of magnifying devices, lights, and other items may be available in your ophthalmologist's office for tryout. If some are found to be useful, he or she can give you a prescription for the type of device and a source where it can be obtained. Some of the higher quality and more useful types of aids may need a prescription and may not be generally available. However, many optical aids are available locally. An extensive collection can be found at the New York Association for the Blind. In order to obtain aids from there, a prescription may be required. A catalog is also available.

The New York Association for the Blind
111 East 59th Street
New York, New York 10022
Telephone: (212) 355-2200

Library Services. Large-print books and recorded books and magazines are available free. The rationale here is that sighted taxpayers have access to the public library, which is free, and if an individual cannot see well enough to read, this material should still be available free in another, more usable form. A special edition of *Books in Print,* entitled *Large Type Books in Print,* lists books that are available in larger-size typefaces. It is, appropriately, printed in large-type print. This catalog may be available in a public library or it can be ordered from

R. R. Bowker Company
Order Department
1180 Avenue of the Americas
New York, New York 10036
Telephone: (212) 764-5100

Local public libraries are a good place to start for large-print publications. Ask the librarian for this sort of material. The Library of Congress has the most extensive collection.

Library of Congress
Division for the Blind and Physically Handicapped
1291 Taylor Street N.W.
Washington, D.C. 20542
Telephone: (202) 882-5500
Toll-free telephone number: (800) 332-5852

The phonograph or tape recorder playback machine is available at the library, also furnished free of charge. It can easily be used by a person with little or no vision. Other sources of such material include the following:

Recording for the Blind, Inc.
215 East 58th Street
New York, New York 10022
Telephone: (212) 751-0860

Choice Magazine Listening
85 Channel Drive
Port Washington, New York 11050
Telephone: (516) 883-8280

Books on Tape, Inc.
Department N
P.O. Box 7900
Newport Beach, California 92660
Toll-free telephone number: (800) 854-6758; in California: (800) 432-7646

Closed circuit television systems for magnification purposes are produced by private companies. They tend to be rather expensive but if they are useful, they may be worth the cost. A closed circuit television system for magnification may be available for tryout at a library. One such company is listed below:

Visualtek
1610 26th Street
Santa Monica, California 90404
Telephone: (213) 829-6841

Specially Adapted Appliances, Tools, and Other Items. One good source of these aids is the American Foundation for the Blind. The main office address is listed below. Many cities have a local office. They publish a catalog entitled *Products for People with Vision Problems.* Samples of some, but usually not nearly all, of these devices may be seen at a local office. Also published by the foundation is a catalog entitled *Directory of Agencies Serving the Visually Handicapped in the U.S.* which is quite extensive and, useful.

American Foundation for the Blind
Customer Service Department
15 West 16th Street
New York, New York 10011
Telephone: (212) 620-2000

More sophisticated devices are also available. Typewriters and calculators exist that pronounce the letters and numbers as the keys are depressed. Even more sophisticated is a reading machine which can convert the printed page into the spoken word. Information can be obtained from

Telesensory Systems, Inc.
3408 Hillview Avenue
P.O. Box 10099
Palo Alto, California 94304
Telephone: (415) 493-2626

Kurzweil Computer Products
33 Cambridge Parkway
Cambridge, Massachusetts 02142
Telephone: (617) 864-4700

Tax Benefits. Depending on the degree of decreased central vision a person has, he or she may be entitled to an income tax deduction or supplementary social security income. One's ophthalmologist can tell if a person qualifies for this exemption and can sign the appropriate forms. The forms are obtainable from your local social security office.

Other Resources. A number of other organizations exist to help people with decreased or absent vision. They are listed as follows.

The National Eye Institute is a good source. This agency has access to much of the information that is available from many places. In addition, this federal agency supports a number of research projects investigating various eye disorders and can provide information about these matters.

National Eye Institute, Information Office
National Institutes of Health
Building 31
Room 6A25
Bethesda, Maryland 20205
Telephone: (301) 496-5248

Information about the rehabilitation of blind people is available from

Office of Human Development Services
Rehabilitation Services Administration
1350 E Street N.W.
Washington, D.C. 20004
Telephone: (202) 727-0518

In addition, each state has a vocational rehabilitation agency.

National Association for Visually Handicapped
3201 Balboa Street
San Francisco, California 94121
Telephone: (415) 221-3201

Information about Braille material is available from a number of institutions. The American Foundation for the Blind, mentioned earlier, can obtain instruction for people in learning to read Braille. The sources listed below, in addition to the Library of Congress are good sources of books printed in Braille.

The Braille Book Bank
422 S. Clinton Avenue
Rochester, New York 14620
Telephone: (716) 232-7770

Instructional Materials Reference Center
American Printing House for the Blind
1839 Frankfurt Avenue
P.O. Box 6085
Louisville, Kentucky 40206
Telephone: (502) 895-2405

The Jewish Braille Institute of America, Inc.
110 East 30th Street
New York, New York 10016
Telephone: (212) 889-2525

Xavier Society for the Blind
The National Catholic Press
and Library for the Visually Handicapped
154 East 23rd Street
New York, New York 10010
Telephone: (212) 473-7800

John Milton Society for the Blind
(represents Protestant Churches)
Room 832
475 Riverside Drive
New York, New York 10115
Telephone: (212) 870-3335

The Howe Press
Perkins School for the Blind
Watertown, Massachusetts 02172
Telephone: (617) 924-3434

Clovernook Home and School for the Blind
7000 Hamilton Avenue
Cincinnati, Ohio 45231
Telephone: (513) 522-3860

Braille Institute
741 North Vermont Avenue
Los Angeles, California 90029
Telephone: (213) 663-1111

Other sources of information, including organizations that provide seeing eye dogs and train people in their use, are listed below:

The Hadley School for the Blind
700 Elm Street
P.O. Box 299
Winnetka, Illinois 60093
Telephone: (312) 446-8111

Veterans Administration
810 Vermont Ave. N.W.
Washington, D.C. 20420
Telephone: (202) 393-4120

A local Veterans Hospital would be the best place to start.

The Delta Gamma Foundation
3250 Riverside Drive
Columbus, Ohio 43221
Telephone: (614) 481-8169

Guide Dogs for the Blind, Inc.
350 Los Ranchitos Road
P.O. Box 1200
San Rafael, California 94915
Telephone: (415) 479-4000

Pilot Dogs, Inc.
625 W. Town Street
Columbus, Ohio 43215
Telephone: (614) 221-6367

Guide Dog Foundation for the Blind, Inc.
109-19 72nd Avenue
Forest Hills, New York 11375
Telephone: (212) 263-4885

International Guiding Eyes, Inc.
2221 Empire Avenue
Burbank, California 91504
Telephone: (213) 849-5439

Leader Dogs for the Blind
1039 South Rochester Road
Rochester, Michigan 48063
Telephone: (313) 651-9011

Guiding Eyes for the Blind
250 East Hartsdale Avenue
Hartsdale, New York 10530
Telephone: (914) 723-2223

The Seeing Eye, Inc.
Morristown, New Jersey 07960
Telephone: (201) 539-4425

RETINAL DETACHMENT AND VITREOUS FLOATERS

The *retina* is a thin tissue that lines the back of the eye and consists mostly of nerves. It is about as thick as a piece of tissue paper and has about 1 million nerves in each eye. These individual nerves are combined into one bundle called the *optic nerve.* The optic nerve leaves the back of the eye and makes connections with nerves in the brain.

Most of the inside of the eye is filled with a material called *vitreous.* In younger people, this vitreous pushes the retina against the back of the eye and thus helps to keep it in position. The vitreous is mostly water, has the consistency of semisoft gelatin, and is perfectly clear in younger people.

Vitreous Floaters

As a person gets older, changes occur in the vitreous and retina. The vitreous becomes less firm and starts to contract away from the retina. Most of it becomes more liquid but some small parts can condense and become more solid. These particles are termed *vitreous floaters.* The floaters reflect light and so their shadows are seen by the patient as black spots. Since the vitreous is more liquid than it once was, these small solid parts move more freely in the vitreous. When the eye is moved to try to focus on them they also move, since they are still somewhat fixed in position, and the vitreous moves when the eye moves. Generally, vitreous floaters appear as small dots or wiggly lines that tend to float in the field of vision. The vitreous does not regenerate or replace itself. This is different from the aqueous in the front of the eye, which was discussed earlier. A vitreous floater can be quite alarming if it is not understood, as the following case shows:

Case 29

Robert B. was a 45-year-old man who had never before worn glasses. He came to me complaining of blurred vision when he did his work as a draftsman. It appeared that he would need reading glasses.

As the examination progressed Robert told me that he also had another problem that he had never told anyone else about. He said that he was afraid everyone would say he was crazy. He was quite agitated and had obviously been quite worried. He said that sometimes he saw spots before his eyes that are like hairs floating on water. He would try to look at the spots and the spots would jump away to the side. He was sure that seeing spots was a sign of being crazy and so he had been afraid to tell anyone, especially his wife, about the problem.

To me, it sounded like the symptoms of a vitreous floater. After a full examination, including dilation of his eyes to check the periphery of his retina and inspection of his vitreous, I decided he had vitreous floaters. I talked with him about these vitreous floaters and also about retinal detachment. Robert seemed much relieved and after he received his reading glasses he told me he finally had a good night's sleep for the first time in months. I encouraged him not to wait so long next time to ask about things that bothered him.

Retinal Detachment

Eventually the vitreous completely separates from the retina. If this happens all at once, no problem generally occurs. However, if a small strand remains attached to the retina, it may pull a small piece of retina with it, thus creating a small hole in the retina. Fluid from the center of the eye can go through this hole and get between the retina and the back of the eye. Enough fluid can get into this place to push the retina out of position. This is then called a *retinal detachment* and occurs in about 2 out of every 1000 people.

A hole in the retina can be caused by other means as well. For example, a traumatic blow or foreign body inside the eye can also cause a hole. After a cataract operation there is a somewhat higher incidence of retinal detachment, about 2 in every 100 people. A variety of causes for this are thought possible, such as trauma during surgery, or simply the shock of decreasing the intraocular pressure by opening the eye, or the fact that there is now more room for the vitreous to move about in after the lens has been removed. Other people, such as those who are extremely myopic, also have a somewhat higher than normal incidence of retinal detachment. Degeneration of parts of the retina can lead to thinning of the retina and is yet another cause of hole formation. Not every hole is large enough or in a position such that fluid can leak through it easily enough to cause a detached retina. Sometimes it is recommended that if the retina is still attached and a hole is found, that treatment with heat (laser) or cold (cryotherapy) be tried. Either of these modalities tends to stimulate formation of a scar around the hole and this scar is then connected to the back lining of the eye. The chances of fluid going through the hole and causing a retinal detachment are thus reduced. A retinal hole or a retinal detachment is not caused by such things as overuse of the eyes, improper glasses, eye strain, or anxiety.

Symptoms of a detached retina are mainly the sensation of a curtain or shadow coming down over the field of vision, or coming up into the field of vision. If the detachment is extensive enough to cover up or include the part of the retina that provides central vision (the macular area), a large reduction in visual acuity may also be noticed. In addition, many sparks, like a Fourth of July fireworks display, may be seen. The sparks are generally rather dramatic. If a blood vessel is torn when the retina detaches, the patient may notice black spots or an enlarging inkblot appearance. Vitreous floaters by themselves are *not* characteristic of a retinal detachment, but because they suggest that the vitreous may be starting to separate from the retina they can be associated with a retinal detachment. For this reason, it is important for a person with vitreous floaters to realize what the symptoms of a retinal detachment are and to have a proper examination. Some sparks or small light flashes may be noticed if the vitreous takes longer than a few seconds to separate from the retina. This is from stretching the nerves of the retina, which leads to a visual sensation. Usually a person does not notice the vitreous separation since it usually happens so fast, or perhaps while sleeping. It is not possible for a patient to be sure, by himself, if he had a normal vitreous separation or a retinal detachment. It is also not possible for a patient to be sure by himself if vitreous floaters are in fact vitreous floaters or are really pigment debris or blood.

Since the success rate in repairing a detached retina is higher if it is repaired soon after it occurs, it is important that a person be seen by an ophthalmologist within one or two days after first noticing symptoms. In other words, it isn't necessary to be seen in a few minutes but the examination should *not* be put off for even one week. If a person is out of town, a local ophthalmologist should be consulted rather than awaiting the return home. The following case illustrates how easy it can be to ignore a serious problem:

Case 30

Tom R. was a man in his fifties who had a family history of cataracts. His mother and grandmother had each had significant cataracts at this age, so when he needed an operation he was optimistic, albeit resigned. He had a cataract operation in each eye spaced several months apart and recovered quite well. He adapted easily to the use of soft contact lenses.

About a year after the operations Tom began to have multiple family problems. His father was in and out of the hospital for treatment of cancer. His wife lost her job when budget cuts occurred. His youngest daughter had several boyfriends whom he didn't think were appropriate.

About this time he also began noticing a blurriness of vision from his left eye. He kept meaning to make an appointment to get his contact lenses checked but he was too preoccupied with other problems. Tom was sure the blurred vision was caused by some debris on the lens that was hard to remove. Since the lenses were about a year old he thought they might even need to be replaced and he really didn't want to spend the money just then. Finally on a Friday afternoon about three weeks later Tom went to his doctor who referred him to me.

I examined him and found that he had a significant retinal detachment in that eye. He underwent surgery the next day and several months later had vision nearly as good as he had before the incident occurred. Tom has since talked with other people who also had retinal detachments and is quite aware of how lucky he was to have had a successful repair after a three-week history. I think Tom will seek help sooner if he notices a problem with the other eye.

Vitreous floaters are initially a troublesome symptom but most people learn to ignore them after they understand what they are. Since this is an ongoing process, it is possible to develop additional floaters at a later time and people generally learn to ignore these as well. It is quite important for people with vitreous floaters to understand the differences between symptoms of more of the same and retinal detachment. If a detached retina is not repaired it will continue to detach and total blindness in that eye will result. A detached retina almost never reattaches by itself.

Repair of a Retinal Detachment. Surgery is necessary in order to repair a detached retina. Prior to surgery an extensive examination of the retina is performed in order to locate all holes or tears in the retina and the precise location of the detached area. A drawing of these findings is generally made. Both the indirect ophthalmoscope and three-mirror lens (see Chapter 1) are used for this examination, which can sometimes take several hours. The side of the eye is also gently indented in order to see the edges of the retina. This technique is called *scleral depression.* Sometimes a technique using ultrasound waves is employed, for example, if significant bleeding has also occurred. The other eye is also examined carefully at this time and in the future since a person who has had a retinal detachment in one eye is more likely to have one in the other eye. However, many people do not have retinal detachments in each eye, so undue concern is unwarranted.

The procedure is usually performed under general anesthesia and takes about three hours. The technique involves buttressing the area that is detached with silicone sponges and/or a plastic encircling band so that the hole is closed; sometimes the fluid behind the retina is drained out. These materials are sewn onto the outside of the eye, are generally not visible after the operation, usually cause no discomfort after the swelling subsides, and are generally left in permanently. In addition, cryotreatment (cold) or diathermy (heat) is given to stimulate scar formation to help keep the retina in the proper position. The eye is rotated in the orbit during these procedures. It is not removed from the head. Both eyes may be covered before and after surgery for a few days to minimize eye movement, which might keep the retina from settling into position.

The present success rate in repairing an uncomplicated retinal detachment is about 80 to 90 percent compared to perhaps 10 percent or less 25 years ago. Complicated retinal detachments include, among others, such things as large holes, large amounts of retina detached, a long period between diagnosis and treatment, or other problems with the eye, such as complications from diabetes or scar tissue formation in the vitreous. Scar tissue can pull on the retina and keep the retina from settling into the proper position. A procedure called a *vitrectomy* may be needed to cut some of these so-called traction bands. Sometimes there are multiple holes and not all of them are located or closed in the first operation and a second operation is needed. Other failures are caused by such things as infection of the buttressing materials, formation of scar tissue in the wrong place that continues to detach the retina, and bleeding, which can also lead to scar tissue formation in the wrong place. These problems may not occur until several months after surgery. A different pair of glasses or a contact lens is generally needed after the operation and it takes several months for all the swelling to subside and for as full a recovery as possible to occur. Even if the retina is successfully reattached, the nerves must begin functioning normally for good vision to result.

The longer a reattached retina stays in proper position, the better the chance for a permanent cure. While the results for retinal detachment surgery may not be quite as certain as they are for cataract surgery, for example, the overall results are good enough that if a detached retina occurs an optimistic, hopeful outlook is realistic.

CHAPTER 6

General Eye Problems

BLOOD VESSELS

Since the eye is a living tissue, it requires various nutrients to survive. These nutrients are carried and distributed, for the most part, by an elaborate system of blood vessels. Nutrients from various sources are dissolved in the blood and the blood is pumped through the circulatory system. The nutrients are removed in various locations as they are needed. Blood flow is actually quite rapid, a full circulation generally taking considerably less than one minute.

Blood vessels carrying blood away from the heart are called *arteries* and those returning blood to the heart are called *veins*. The large arteries branch into smaller arteries and finally into the smallest blood vessels, called *capillaries*. The capillaries are connected with the small veins which connect to the larger veins. The largest vessels, as a rough estimate, are about one-quarter inch in diameter, whereas the capillaries cannot be seen without a microscope since they are barely wide enough for a red blood cell to fit through.

A blockage or a partial blockage can occur in any blood vessel for a number of reasons. Some causes include blood clots, a piece of calcium released from another location, a gradual narrowing of the lumen of the vessel that finally completely closes, or spasm of the muscles around the vessel. Depending on where and how long such an occlusion of blood flow occurs, one has a greater or lesser problem. An occlusion in a remote capillary that lasts less than one second may not even be noticed. A sudden permanent occlusion in a large vessel can cause severe problems and even death.

In the eye the large artery that supplies the nerves in the back of the eye (retina) sometimes becomes completely blocked. This is called a *central retinal artery occlusion.* Sometimes there is enough force behind the blockage to reopen the vessel. If this happens fast enough, there may be little damage, but generally this is a serious problem and severe visual loss occurs. The eye can live without a blood supply for only a short time without suffering permanent damage.

The symptoms of a central retinal artery occlusion are sudden, total loss of vision in the affected eye. Sometimes breathing into a paper bag helps. This is because the carbon dioxide content of the blood may be increased by this technique, and since increased carbon dioxide leads to dilation of blood vessels, the central retinal artery and other vessels may be dilated enough to allow the obstructing material to pass through. Sometimes, as mentioned earlier, massaging the eye will push the obstructing material along. Contact an ophthalmologist immediately if you have these symptoms, since some diseases of the blood vessels, such as temporal arteritis, can be treated with medication hopefully to prevent the same problem in the other eye. In some cases, it may even be possible to retain some vision in the affected eye if the occlusion is not complete or does not last too long.

A more common event is blockage of a smaller vein in the retina, called a *branch vein occlusion.* Depending on the location, the final visual result may be satisfactory. If the blockage lasts a long time, nearby vessels may expand to compensate and new vessels may actually form. When new vessels form, problems can develop because these new vessels are not normal and they tend to leak. Sometimes laser therapy is useful in treating this problem.

There is no definite way to prevent problems from developing with the blood vessels, but many things are thought to help. These were outlined in Chapter 1, but are briefly mentioned again here. Adequate exercise and a good diet are important. When the blood vessels become coated with large amounts of fat, for example, the lumen may become narrower and partial or complete occlusion can occur more easily. Exercise is thought to help remove some of these fat deposits. Moderating one's intake of fatty food is also thought to be of help. Your family physician can discuss this in more detail and can measure certain fats in the blood, such as cholesterol, to help monitor the situation.

Medical problems, such as high blood pressure and diabetes mellitus, can also affect the blood vessels. Problems with the blood itself may cause difficulties. For example, the blood may be too thick or, as in sickle cell disease, sickled blood cells may occlude the vessels. These problems and others should be watched for and treated, if possible, by your family doctor.

Many other problems can occur with the blood vessels. Most are not common. However, one particular condition called *retrolental fibroplasia* (RLF) can occur in babies who are born prematurely, and can cause severe problems in the eye. In this disease the blood vessels at the edge of the retina form improperly and various problems result, such as leakage, scarring, and decreased vision. Newer techniques of treatment of premature babies in the nursery have reduced the incidence and severity of complications of this condition.

BLEEDING

Subconjunctival Hemorrhage

It is important to distinguish bleeding on the outside of the eye from bleeding on the inside of the eye. The medical term for bleeding is *hemorrhage.* One type of bleeding on the outside of the eye is called a *subconjunctival hemorrhage.* This problem can occur for a number of reasons. The most common cause is trauma, as when one is struck near the eye by a ball or a fist. However, it is also common to have such a problem if one rubs the eye too hard or sneezes particularly hard or severely strains when moving the bowels.

The white part of the eye is a relatively thick, tough tissue, called *sclera.* It is covered by a tissue called the *conjunctiva.* The conjunctiva is about as thick as a piece of facial tissue. Just beneath this tissue is a somewhat thicker tissue called *Tenon's capsule,* which also covers the white part of the eye. In the front part of the eye, the conjunctiva and Tenon's capsule are attached to each other and to the sclera at the place where the white part of the eye and the colored part (iris) come together. This location is called the *limbus.* In all other places there is a small space between the conjunctiva and Tenon's capsule. This space is normally filled with a watery fluid. Blood vessels are located in and beneath Tenon's capsule.

If a small blood vessel breaks for any of the reasons listed above, a few drops of blood may become trapped between Tenon's capsule and the conjunctiva. The conjunctiva is often strong enough to prevent the blood from dripping over the lid but the blood can spread between the conjunctiva and Tenon's capsule, and if there is enough bleeding, the whole white part of the eye may appear red as it is covered with blood. More often, only a few drops of blood leak from a damaged blood vessel before the opening is closed by a clot. These few drops, however, can gradually spread around in the space between the conjunctiva and Tenon's capsule, much as a drop of water can spread between two pieces of waxed paper. This is why what initially appears to be only a small bleed can in a few days look like it is more severe. Rubbing the eye spreads the blood even more.

Sometimes the blood in a subconjunctival hemorrhage is not free-flowing and it gets trapped in the meshwork of Tenon's capsule. It can then appear as a bubble of blood. Vision is usually not adversely affected.

A subconjunctival hemorrhage takes longer than one might think to resolve. Usually at least two weeks and frequently two months are needed for total resolution. This is because the blood does not flow out, but must actually be degraded and transported out by various cells. Degradation products may make it appear yellow after a few days. This is not a cause for concern. A similar observation can be made of a bruise on the leg, for example. The bruise changes colors as the blood from broken blood vessels is degraded and removed.

Hyphema

Bleeding inside the eye is quite different. It may occur in the front (*hyphema*) or the back (*vitreous hemorrhage*) of the eye. Bleeding in the front part is discussed first. This type appears over the colored part (iris) of the eye and may be quite small and difficult for an untrained observer to see. The blood is actually in the anterior chamber, that is, the space between the iris and the back of the cornea. Vision is usually fairly normal if the hyphema is small. It generally layers out to form a reddish-black area at the bottom of the eye. A hyphema can, however, be much larger and fill the entire anterior chamber. In this case, vision would be severely reduced.

There are several reasons why this condition is more serious, even though it looks to most people as if it would be less serious. The eye is a closed compartment and even a small amount of blood can raise the pressure in the eye enough to cause damage to the nerves. In addition, a small amount of blood can clog up the channels that normally allow the watery fluid in the eye to circulate. This can also raise the intraocular pressure.

Furthermore, such bleeding has a tendency to rebleed in a small number of cases. Rebleeding tends to be in larger amounts and thus potentially more serious. The greatest chance of a recurrent bleed is three to five days after the initial event. Subconjunctival hemorrhage and hyphema can occur simultaneously.

Vitreous Hemorrhage

Bleeding farther back inside the eye in the material called vitreous is called a vitreous hemorrhage. A vitreous hemorrhage is generally not visible to a casual observer, although the vision of the patient is usually decreased. A hyphema or vitreous hemorrhage is usually associated with severe trauma to the eye or abnormal blood vessels, such as might be found in diabetes mellitus or bleeding problems such as hemophilia, or other causes.

Frequently a hyphema or a vitreous hemorrhage that is caused by trauma will resolve without permanent complications if there has been no damage to other structures of the eye. However, sometimes it is necessary to surgically remove the blood. A hyphema may resolve in a few days but a vitreous hemorrhage may take several months. Bedrest with both eyes patched to minimize movement may be recommended, depending on the severity of the bleeding. If the bleeding is caused by another problem, an effort is made to try to correct or control that problem, if possible, to prevent a recurrence.

INFECTIONS

Infections can occur on the outside or inside of the eye, as in any other part of the body. There are a number of mechanisms or barriers that normally prevent infections from progressing. For example, tears wash away much debris with each blink. In addition, normal tears have various components that kill or inactivate various organisms.

The most common organisms that can cause infections on or in the eye are bacteria and viruses. Bacteria are quite small organisms composed of only one cell. They vary in their nutritional requirements and other environmental needs. For example, some grow well only in the presence of much oxygen and others grow well only if there is very little oxygen surrounding them. Viruses are much smaller and are more dependent on other cells or organisms to supply their nutritional needs. Most bacteria are susceptible to antibiotic drugs but very few viruses are. Names of some common bacteria are Staphylococci, Streptococci, and *Pseudomonas.* Common viruses are herpes simplex, herpes zoster, adenoviruses, enteroviruses, and the trachoma-inclusion conjunctivitis (TRIC) group of organisms, which fall inbetween viruses and bacteria.

Other types of organisms that can cause infections are called fungi and protozoa. A fungus is somewhat more complex than a bacteria and a protozoa is even more complex. Fungal infections are not very common in colder climates, but they are seen in areas that are more hot and humid and in all areas in people who do not have normal resistance to infection. However, even then they are rare. Examples of fungi that can cause infections are *Candida* and *Aspergillus.* An example of a protozoan infection that is occasionally seen is toxoplasmosis. There are drugs available that can be used to treat most fungal and protozoal infections.

Conjunctivitis

Infections on the outside of the eye are somewhat less worrisome than those inside, but all should be taken seriously and treated by a physician. Conjunctivitis is the name for an inflammation, frequently caused by an infection, affecting the conjunctiva. The conjunctiva is a thin tissue that lies over the white part (sclera) of the eye. A patient with conjunctivitis may note a mild, intermittent discomfort or there may be more severe pain and sensitivity to light. There may be a discharge and the eyelids may be stuck together in the morning by dried discharge. Most commonly a bacteria or a virus will affect this area. Bacteria are normally found on a person's skin and sometimes it is this bacterial species that causes the conjunctivitis. Generally, in this case there are predisposing factors. For example, there may be decreased tear secretion and the conjunctiva gets somewhat dried out. It is then not able to resist the infection as well as it used to. At other times, excessive wind or sun exposure may cause a similar problem. Sometimes merely exposure to the organisms in the air will cause it. Contaminated makeup is another common cause. If makeup is used and conjunctivitis occurs, makeup use should be stopped and the bottles discarded. After the problem is resolved fresh preparations should be purchased if permission is given to resume makeup use.

Conjunctivitis should be considered contagious. This means that it can be transferred generally by hand-to-eye contact, from eye to eye and person to person. If any type of infection of or around the eye is present, precautions to minimize its spread should be exercised, for example, care should be taken not to use the towels that other people use nor should other people use the towels that the infected person uses.

Antibiotic drops are generally prescribed for bacterial conjunctivitis. The technique of eye drop application is discussed in Chapter 1. Frequently, they are also prescribed for viral infections to try to prevent other bacteria from starting to grow, since the viral infection makes the conjunctiva less able to resist other infections. These drops are generally used at least four times a day and frequently eight times. Generally, they should be used for at least seven days and often 10 days or more to completely eliminate all the organisms.

The eyelids should be kept clean with moist tissues, or as directed. Usually the symptoms will subside much sooner, but if the drops are stopped sooner there is a tendency for the infection to recur. If there is a predisposing cause, such as from the use of contaminated makeup, or decreased tear production, it is also necessary to try to treat this as well. Drops and ointments should be discarded after use and not reused for a subsequent episode. They too may be contaminated or outdated.

Other viral infections, such as some of those causing the common cold or diarrhea, can also cause a viral conjunctivitis. These usually clear up when the main infection resolves.

Not all inflammations of the conjunctiva are caused by infectious agents. An allergy to dust or pollen or makeup can also cause conjunctivitis. Treatment in this case would consist of trying to remove the agent causing the problem (the allergen), and using mild anti-inflammatory drugs such as a mild antihistamine. As mentioned in an earlier section, there are many causes of a red eye. Conjunctivitis is only one of these many causes. Some can be quite serious and ophthalmologic consultation should be obtained in case of any question. The following case illustrates how serious a problem a red eye may actually be:

Case 31

Norman O. was a middle-aged man who had rarely had any problem with his eyes. He wore reading glasses and had had an episode of conjunctivitis a few years earlier. One day he noticed some pain and redness in his right eye. He thought it was another episode of conjunctivitis and tried treating it with some nonprescription eye drops he bought in a drug store. They seemed to help somewhat and when Norman went out into the sun there was still some pain but less than before. That evening the pain started again and he called his local doctor, who prescribed an antibiotic drop. It really didn't help very much. The next day when Norman went outside the pain was less but still present. That night he went to a movie and the pain increased. He used more drops. In the middle of the night the pain became worse and he started vomiting. He tried to wait until the morning to call his doctor. Finally, his wife called the doctor who recommended that he see an ophthalmologist.

He did and was found to have acute narrow-angle glaucoma, a

relatively rarer form of glaucoma. Various medications and drops were given. He was told that the entrances to the drainage channels in his eyes were narrower than normal. When he was in a darker place, the pupil enlarged and closed the drainage channels to fluid leaving his eye. When he went into the sun, the pupil constricted and the drainage channels were not as closed. Thus, the pressure inside his eye was higher and the pain was more severe when he was in a room with less light. Since the pressure was still too high, even in the bright sun, Norman had some pain, but not as much, when he went outside.

After his condition stabilized, Norman underwent a surgical procedure to provide an alternate pathway for the fluid to leave his eye. A few months later he had the same procedure done on his other eye so that he would not have the same problem with it. Norman has not had any further difficulty and is quite certain he will seek ophthalmologic care more quickly if he should ever have another problem with his eye. He feels fortunate that permanent damage, such as scar formation or damage to the nerves in his eye, did not occur.

Eyelid Infections

Infections can also occur in the skin of the eyelids. These infections are also potentially quite serious since the organisms can travel into blood vessels that connect directly with the brain. Antibiotic pills, lid scrubs, and hot compresses may be needed. This problem is discussed further in Chapter 4.

Infections of the Cornea

Infections that occur on the cornea are very serious. The cornea is the clear tissue that covers the colored part (iris) of the eye. In this case, if a bacterial infection is suspected, it is usually necessary to take a sample of these organisms and grow them (culture them) in the laboratory in order to analyze them and find out which antibiotics to use. Drops may be given every half hour and injections of antibiotics around the area may also be needed. The reason these infections are so serious is that the bacteria can quickly erode through to the inside of the eye. Bacteria generally double in number about every 20 to 40 minutes so it is important to treat these infections quickly and completely. In addition, scarring of the cornea may result from a prolonged infection and may lead to reduced vision.

Viral infections can also occur in the cornea. One of the common ones is the herpes simplex virus. This virus also causes the common "cold sore" which may occur on the lips, for example. Fortunately, new drugs are available to help treat this condition. Herpes simplex infections can also cause scarring and may recur. Herpes zoster is the virus that causes chicken pox. It can cause problems on the cornea as a result of its growth on the skin of the lids and in the nerves. This can lead to drying of the cornea because of a decreased blink reflex. This virus infection may also recur, particularly during stressful periods. Trachoma is probably the most common eye infection in the world; however, it is not so common in the United States. Trachoma is *not* the same as glaucoma. It can be treated, but frequently recurs and causes scarring of both the cornea and the eyelids. It is contagious and is seen in dry, dusty climates where shortages of water make it difficult to prevent the spread from person to person. Hand-to-eye transmission is common, since hands and towels cannot be adequately cleaned.

Infections Inside the Eye

Infections inside the eye itself (*endophthalmitis*) are the most serious. When bacteria grow they produce pus and scarring. There is very little room inside the eye for this extra material and the intraocular pressure can increase. In addition, this material is quite harmful to the nerves in the back of the eye. Cultures are necessary and antibiotics may be injected directly into the eye; sometimes an instrument is used to remove much of this material. This type of infection generally only occurs when the normal barriers of defense are not intact. For example, after an operation on the eye where an opening is actually made and then sewn closed, infection can occur if the wound is not completely closed, if it reopens, or if organisms were introduced when the wound was open during surgery. Fortunately, this complication of eye surgery is quite rare. Another cause of this type of infection is trauma. It is also seen in people who are on medications that reduce their ability to resist infections. Fortunately, the incidence of endophthalmitis is quite low. Recent techniques have somewhat improved the prognosis, which used to be quite poor.

Some infections inside the eye can follow a course that may flare up from time to time. After treatment of these flare-up episodes, long periods of quiescence may occur. However, scarring can occur during these flare-up episodes and it is more of a problem if it occurs in some areas of the eye than in others. Examples are toxoplasmosis and histoplasmosis.

Infections occurring during fetal life can also cause problems with the eye, ranging from mild to severe. For example, the rubella (measles) virus can cause problems in eye development. The severity of a given infection depends on when during gestation the infection occurs and on the type of infectious agent.

CHRONIC INFLAMMATIONS

There are a number of diseases that tend to wax and wane, that is, they get better, then they get worse some time later, and then they may get better again. The periods when they are better are called *remissions* and when they are worse are termed *recurrences.* Frequently it is never known, even after an extensive investigation, what is causing the problem in the first place, although there are many theories. Other times the cause is known. Even though the exact cause is not known, however, the symptoms and effects may often be controllable. Since these diseases tend to occur for long periods of time, often years, they are called *chronic.* However, sometimes the periods of remission may last years so that it seems like a full cure has taken place and sometimes they may even stop recurring.

Diseases in this category are usually inflammations, that is, there is an irritation that causes what is called an *inflammatory response.* An inflammatory response consists of certain characteristics, among which is the presence of certain small cells. These cells, which in other parts of the body are helpful, can sometimes cause damage in a tissue like the eye. For example, a scar in the skin is fine, but a scar over the central retina is not so good since the nerve cells in that area would no longer function. A scar over the aqueous outflow channels could lead to glaucoma. Thus, treatment of these diseases often includes drugs that inhibit these cells. Such drugs are called anti-inflammatory drugs. Some of these are potent drugs and must be used under medical supervision.

Examples of such chronic inflammatory diseases include chronic iritis, chronic uveitis, scleritis, and recurrent optic neuritis. Iritis, uveitis, scleritis, and optic neuritis can, however, occur as one-time episodes that do not recur. Iritis means inflammation of the iris. Uveitis means inflammation of the uvea. The uvea is composed of the iris, ciliary body, and choroid (blood vessels near the retina). Scleritis is inflammation of the sclera. Optic neuritis is inflammation of the optic nerve. Other parts of the eye can also have an inflammation and would be similarly named. Inflammations of the eye may be associated with other diseases that may affect other parts of the body, for example, rheumatoid arthritis and sarcoid. Various drugs and toxins can also cause inflammations, for example, methyl alcohol.

The symptoms of these different diseases may vary widely. Some people have marked decrease in vision, while others have only a mild decrease. In some of these diseases, some people may have deep, aching pain in their eye, while others have little or no pain. A disease such as iritis may be confused with conjunctivitis, for example, by an inexperienced observer. Iritis is treated differently from conjunctivitis and if it is not treated properly, undesirable scarring can occur. This is one reason why even a seemingly trivial problem should be properly evaluated.

TUMORS

In simple terms a tumor is a mass of tissue growing in an uncontrolled manner. Such a tumor may remain small and not spread. This type is called a *benign* tumor. A *malignant* tumor, on the other hand, may grow more rapidly and can spread to other parts of the body. Fortunately, a malignant tumor, commonly known as cancer, is rare in the eye. There are, however, a few that do occur. It is important to try to diagnose them before they become advanced, since treatment in the early stages is generally more effective and may even result in a cure.

Such a tumor can occur on the eyelids; these tumors can frequently be completely removed without too much difficulty if they are diagnosed and treated early. In the later stages these tumors can spead into vital areas such as the brain, making complete removal not really possible. Lid tumors have been mistaken for chalazia, but unlike a chalazion, a tumor does not regress. A biopsy can confirm the diagnosis. A biopsy means taking a small sample of the lesion and looking at it under the microscope for certain characteristics. Suspicious lesions of the lids are generally biopsied, if possible, to see whether there is a tumor or not, and if so, what type. Appropriate therapy can then be administered.

Other tumors can occur inside the eyeball itself. These tumors may originate in different parts of the eye. For example, a retinoblastoma originates in cells of the retina and an angioma originates in cells of the blood vessels. These can be quite serious. However, if they are diagnosed early, visual loss may be confined to the one eye only. In a later state some tumors may spread to other parts of the body and to the other eye, and can even result in death.

When these tumors have spread they are much more difficult to treat. Often malignant tumors inside the eye grow quite slowly and look similar to benign ones, that is, not serious tumors. Thus, frequent examinations and photographs may be used initially, instead of a more radical treatment.

Tumors can also occur in the brain itself and interfere with the nerves coming from the eye to the area of the brain where visual information is processed. A number of techniques are available to diagnose and treat these tumors. For example, sometimes changes in the visual field are noted since, depending on its location, the tumor may interfere just with nerves that serve one part of the field. In other cases the optic nerve may appear swollen. Headaches are rarely caused by such tumors, but visual symptoms of various sorts may be noted.

Sometimes tumors in other parts of the body can spread to the eye. However, this usually occurs in a later stage of such a disease. Treatment varies, depending on the nature and extent of the tumor, both in the eye and elsewhere.

An ophthalmologist is trained to diagnose and treat these various tumors. Frequently, other physicians are involved in the care of people with tumors. You should not hesitate to obtain another opinion if there is any question in your mind about the proposed diagnosis or treatment. In fact, frequently your ophthalmologist will request that you be evaluated by another physician. In this case he would generally refer you to a specific physician or give you a choice of physicians to see.

Many of these tumors turn out to be benign, of which a nevus is a common example. Thus, one should not be unduly apprehensive.

DIABETES MELLITUS

Diabetes mellitus is a disease that may affect the small blood vessels, called capillaries, throughout the body, to varying degrees in different people. Since these blood vessels also supply the eye with oxygen and other materials, it is not surprising that sometimes people with diabetes develop problems with their eyes. Some of these problems are the same type of problem that anyone else can develop, although they may manifest themselves somewhat earlier. For example, people with diabetes have a somewhat higher incidence and somewhat earlier occurrence of cataract formation than the general population. The treatment of this problem, however, is essentially the same as for the general population. See Chapter 4 for a full discussion of the problem of cataracts.

Other problems are more unique to the disease process of diabetes. For example, if the amount of sugar in the blood changes by a large amount, such as when the disease is not well controlled, the amount of sugar in the lens inside the eye also changes. This leads to swelling of the lens, since more water is absorbed into the lens to balance the amount of sugar. This swollen lens has a different power and a patient with this problem may notice blurred vision. The sugar does not flow out of the lens as easily as it flowed in because it is converted to a different compound and this compound does not flow out as fast. Thus, after an episode of poor control of diabetes it takes considerably longer for the refraction to stabilize than for the amount of sugar in the blood to stabilize. It may take several weeks for the refraction to stabilize; after it does stabilize the original eyeglasses may again be appropriate.

Some people who have had diabetes for many years (at least 10 or 15) develop growth of new capillaries (*neovascularization*) to supply various parts of their eye that are being inadequately supplied (see Fig. 26 A,B). What on first glance may seem to be a beneficial devel-

FIGURE 26A, B. Neovascularization. These are examples of the sort of abnormal new vessels that can occur in patients with diabetes mellitus.

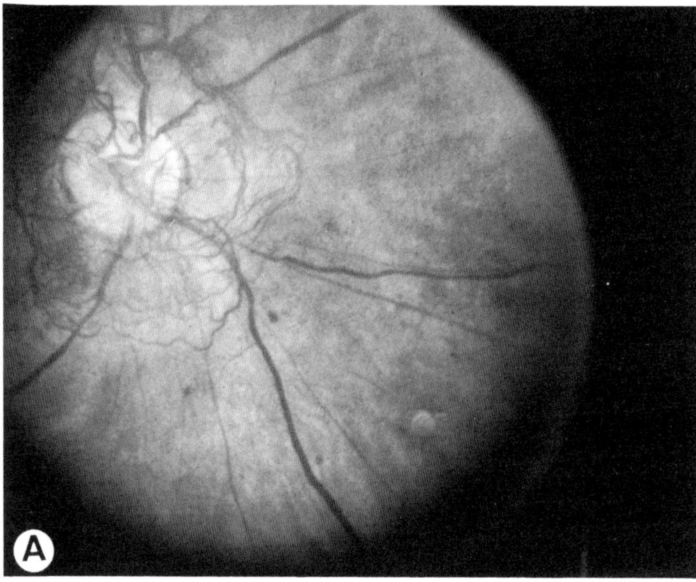

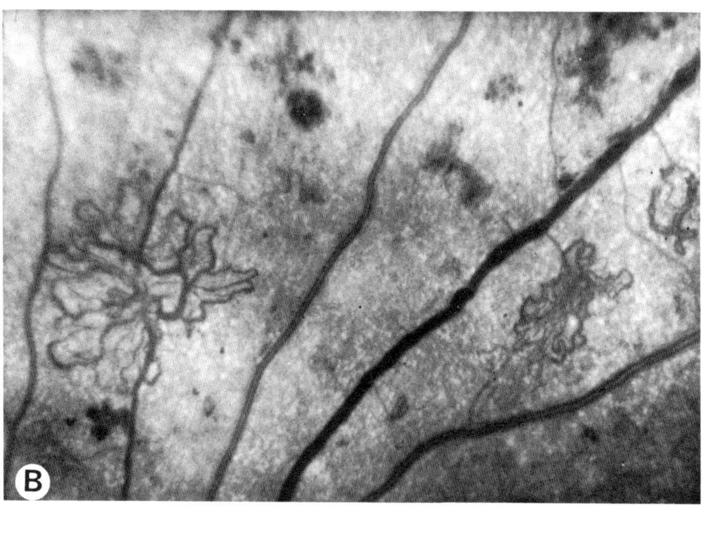

opment frequently turns out not to be because of the location and type of new vessels formed. These vessels may grow into abnormal locations, for example, and block the drainage channels for the fluid that fills the inside of the eye. Since this fluid is produced by glands inside the eye, increased pressure (glaucoma) can result if the fluid cannot drain out at the same rate it enters the eye. The increased pressure can cause damage to the nerves in the back of the eye, the retina. See Chapter 4 for additional information on the problem of glaucoma. These neovascular blood vessels also tend to leak and the subsequent bleeding and scarring can result in total loss of vision.

It is thought that one stimulus for growth of these potentially harmful blood vessels is an area where the tissue is damaged but not dead. If an area of damaged tissue becomes dead, new blood vessels do not tend to grow and complications from them tend not to occur.

Recently, the laser has been used to destroy areas where this damaged tissue may be in the hope of reducing the stimulus for these new blood vessels to form. It is not known for certain why laser treatment works, but in certain cases it is felt to be of significant benefit. These areas that are destroyed are generally small and are off to the side. Usually, there is little if any change in visual acuity after such a treatment. However, if a visual field defect were very carefully looked for (see Chapter 4), one might be seen. This is a small price to pay to hopefully slow down or even prevent total visual loss from a severe bleeding episode. Originally an attempt was made to actually destroy the abnormal blood vessels themselves, but this did not work very well because these vessels frequently started bleeding. In addition, some of the surrounding healthy tissue was damaged and this damaged tissue further stimulated neovascularization.

One way to tell which parts of the eye are damaged is by using photography after injection of a fluorescent dye into the arm. This dye makes it easier to see abnormal blood vessels and other areas of damaged tissue. The technique using photography with a fluorescein dye injection is called *fluorescein angiography.* It is a useful technique in diagnosis and treatment of a number of other disorders of the eye. Depending on the findings of this study, laser treatment may be recommended; however, some types of changes in the retina are not treated with a laser. Laser treatment will *not* improve vision. It may even reduce it slightly because of swelling, for example, from the heat of the laser. The main reason for giving this treatment is to try to prevent or at least to slow down formation of new blood vessels and subsequent bleeding. These problems can lead to total loss of vision in the eye, as mentioned before. This is an important concept to understand before any treatment is administered. The following case describes one patient's experience:

Case 32

Sylvester L. had had diabetes mellitus for many years, with no significant problems. He had regular eye examinations to check for any complications from the diabetes. On one visit his ophthalmologist told him that abnormal new blood vessels were starting to form in various areas of his eyes. Some of them were leaking. Sylvester was told about various potential problems and treatments, one of which involved the use of a laser.

Being an educated, scientific type of businessman, Sylvester was receptive to new ideas and innovations in his business but always tried to carefully investigate any new proposal. He introduced a computer system, for example, after extensive research of which type, model, and manufacturer to use. Thus, it was characteristic of him to want more information about this proposed laser treatment. He read the results of the nationwide multicenter cooperative study sponsored by the National Eye Institute, which investigated the use of the laser in treating this problem. He was impressed by the careful attention to uniform protocols with proper randomization techniques. When he finished his investigation, he decided to have the treatment. He understood that it was not a cure, but he hoped that rapid and severe progression of the problem would be delayed for awhile, as the results of the study suggested would be possible.

Laser treatment may be given in about three or four sessions that each last about 30 minutes per eye, on an outpatient basis. The patient sits at an instrument similar to the slit lamp used in the general eye examination. The eye is dilated first, if possible. The laser beam itself is perceived as a bright light and the amount of pain varies from person to person. Although it is somewhat uncomfortable, it is generally not intolerable. Aspirin should *not* be used to relieve any pain after treatment as it can sometimes cause bleeding. Tylenol or a pain medication prescribed by your ophthalmologist should be used, if needed.

During episodes of bleeding from retinal blood vessels, blood can enter the vitreous and the irritation by the blood can cause scar tissue formation. These vitreous scars can contract and pull the retina out of position and can also be so dense that they block light from getting to the retina.

Recently, a technique has been developed to actually cut vitreous bands and/or vitreous from the inside of the eye. This technique is called a vitrectomy and is a major surgical operation done under general anesthesia. Much of this scarring may be able to be cut or removed so that further complications do not occur. A retinal detachment caused by contraction of this scar tissue is quite difficult to repair and the success rate is not as high as a retinal detachment without these additional problems.

Some people with diabetes have episodes of double vision. This may be caused by poor blood supply to the muscles that move the eyes or to the nerves that control the muscles. Often this problem resolves in a few weeks, but consultation with an ophthalmologist should be obtained if double vision is noted to be sure that there is not another, more serious cause for it.

It is important to realize that *not* everyone with diabetes, even after 20 years or more with the disease, develops these potentially severe problems. Many people have diabetes for 50 years or more with *no* problems at all with their eyes. It is important, however, if a person has diabetes that he be seen on a regular basis by an ophthalmologist, so that any appropriate, available treatment can be discussed and perhaps administered at an early stage in the development of a problem.

TRAUMA

Some information on this topic was discussed in Chapter 1; however, more detailed information on certain topics is given here.

Blowout Fracture

The eyeball is fairly well protected from injury. There are thick bones surrounding most of the globe and these bones form what is called the orbit. A cushion of fat between the globe and bones of the orbit provides additional protection. However, severe trauma can actually break these bones and displace the globe.

One of the more common sites of damage is the bone along the lower rim of the orbit. The part of this bone that is under the globe is somewhat thinner and therefore weaker than other bones. This type of injury is called a blowout fracture. The problem with breaking the bone in this location is that muscles that move the eyeball and nerves that give sensation to this part of the face can become trapped between pieces of bone. Motility and sensation are then reduced.

Much swelling, and frequently, bleeding are associated with this type of trauma. Thus, much of the restriction of motion of the globe may be caused by the swelling. This can result in double vision, which may resolve when the swelling subsides. An x-ray may be taken to determine whether a bone has been broken.

Treatment for this problem is first to test the patient's vision and then examine the eye as much as possible to see if there has been other damage. Frequently there is no significant damage to the eyeball itself. Cold compresses can be applied for the first 24 hours to reduce the swelling.

Surgery is sometimes needed to reposition the broken bones or to release trapped muscles or nerves. The decision when or if to do surgery depends on the degree of swelling, restriction of motion, and loss of sensation. Sometimes no surgical repair is needed. In the interim, if the problem of double vision is too bothersome, a patch may be worn over the affected eye.

Another common fracture site is the bone along the nose. These fractures usually need to be surgically repaired because of the risk of infection and difficulty in breathing.

Injury of the Eyeball

Actual injury to the eyeball itself can also occur. Pieces of metal or glass from grinding or explosions can penetrate or injure the eye. Fortunately, these fragments often do not completely penetrate into the inside of the eye. They may become embedded in the outside layers of the eye and may be extracted without too much difficulty. This is discussed in Chapter 4 in the section on the cornea. Special x-rays may be taken to see if fragments are inside or behind the eye. It is important to be sure that the eye has not been ruptured or perforated, even if the injury appears trivial. An ophthalmologic examination should be obtained for this purpose. If there is any question of actual damage to the eye, care should be taken not to push on the eyeball. A paper cup taped over the eye or a light bandage will protect the eye until help can be obtained.

If these fragments actually cut the eye or penetrate into the inside they must be removed if possible and the cut must be sewn closed. This is usually done in an operating room with the use of a microscope and very fine suture materials. It is important that this be done for a number of reasons. The risk of an infection in an open wound is very great and such an infection can lead to total loss of vision. Depending on the location of the cut, it is even possible for such an infection to spread into the brain. If the foreign material is iron, it can rust, and this is quite damaging to the nerves. Inflammation and scarring can occur. Glaucoma can also occur if there has been traumatic damage to or subsequent scarring of the aqueous outflow channels.

When the cut actually goes through to the inside of the eye, another rather peculiar problem can also develop, called *sympathetic ophthalmia.* Antibodies are made to tissues that are not normally exposed to the cells that make antibodies. These antibodies can then react with the undamaged eye and lead to loss of vision in that eye. For this reason, a badly damaged, nonseeing eye may be removed (enucleated) to try to prevent damage to the remaining normal eye, and also for cosmetic reasons. If the damaged eye retains some useful vision, however, it is often left in place since it is frequently possible to treat sympathetic ophthalmia with medication. It is a very rare disease.

If an eye is removed, artificial ones can be made that in some cases appear quite realistic. The artificial eye is usually a removable plastic shell that is custom-fit and painted. Some mobility of the artificial eye may even be present if the muscles were not too badly damaged. By looking straight ahead and turning the head more, the loss of motion in the prosthesis is not noticed as much by others. Your ophthalmologist can work with you and an ocularist to try to achieve an acceptable cosmetic result. Sometimes surgical revision of the socket may be needed.

Interaction with Blind Persons

If an individual has one eye removed but still has one normal eye certain problems arise. These were discussed in Chapter 2, in the section on depth perception. If both eyes are lost, other considerations are necessary.

Psychiatric consultation will probably be necessary to cope with the emotional problems of the loss of vision. Much help, however, can be provided by friends, relatives, and acquaintances. These people should keep several concepts in mind.

Being blind is not the same as being deaf. There is no need to shout at a blind person if he has normal hearing. When approaching a blind person, identify yourself. Don't expect a blind person to recognize each person's voice (although with practice blind people learn to recognize some people by their voice and even footsteps). Do not pet or otherwise distract a seeing eye dog. If a blind person appears to need help, identify yourself and ask if help is needed. When leaving a blind person, be sure to tell him so. If a blind person needs to be led, it is best for him or her to grasp an outstretched arm and follow the leader rather than being pushed or pulled. The leader should keep talking and give advance warning when stairs, curbs, doorways, and turns are approached. These techniques are also useful in interacting with a person who may be temporarily blind, for example, from patches over each eye for treatment of corneal abrasions.

When speaking to a blind person talk directly to him so that your voice isn't muffled. Directions should be given in terms of the number of blocks, for example, rather than street names. When showing a blind person where to sit, put his hands on the back of the chair or on the seat and let him feel the edges himself. When giving him change tell him which bills are which.

Efforts should be made to integrate blind people into society as much as possible. Overprotection and pity of a blind person, instead of patience and sympathetic understanding, can diminish the individual's sense of self-worth. Adequate exercise is still needed. Treadmills, stationary bicycles, and calisthenics may be appropriate. Thousands of blind individuals are leading useful, productive, relatively independent lives, and that should be the goal. A number of agencies and organizations that may be of help are listed in Chapter 5.

Injury of the Eyelids and Extraocular Muscles

Sometimes the eye and orbital bones are normal but the eyelids are cut, as in a knife wound. It is important to try to repair these wounds since problems can develop if they are not. For example, during a blink the lids actually push tears across the eye in a smooth manner. If the edge of the lid (called the margin) is not smooth the tears are not properly distributed and parts of the eye may get dry, which can lead to irritation and infections. Corneal ulcers and even total loss of vision can occur in such cases. In addition, the tear ducts may have been cut and tears can flow over the lid onto the cheek if they are not repaired satisfactorily. Therefore, it is important to have proper surgical repair of lid problems. In addition, it is important to ascertain that the eye really is normal and that only the lids are affected.

If the muscles that move the lids are damaged, and not adequately repaired, the lids may not close properly and the eye can be severely damaged from drying and infection.

The extraocular muscles, the muscles on the outside of the eye that move the eye from side to side and up and down, can also be damaged by various forms of trauma. Surgical repair of such muscle and lid injuries may be possible as well.

HEREDITARY PROBLEMS

A number of problems relating to the eye are inherited. It is worthwhile to briefly discuss in somewhat simplified terms some of the basic principles of heredity so that some of these problems can be better understood.

A *hereditary disease* is the direct result of a particular genetic composition. A person's genetic composition is the total of his or her various *genes.* Genes control the various developmental and regulatory processes of the body. Some of these processes appear in fetal development, some appear later in life, such as the onset of puberty, and others appear even later, such as certain problems of aging. Hereditary diseases may be seen in some or all members of a family or may skip generations. They may appear only or more often in only males or only females.

A *familial disease* occurs in some or all members of a given family. It may or may not be hereditary or it may be partially hereditary. Environmental factors, such as exposure of the various members of the family to the same toxins, infectious agents, or nutritional deficiences, could also be the cause of a familial disease. Sometimes people in a family may have a hereditary tendency to develop a particular disease, but it only develops if certain environmental factors are also present. Abnormal reactions to certain drugs are an example of this last type of process. In this case, a problem only develops if the individual has the hereditary tendency to have a problem and also happens to be exposed to the particular drug that causes the problem.

A *congenital disease* is a disease that is present at the time of birth. Diseases or processes that are manifested later are said to be *acquired.* Both congenital and acquired diseases may be hereditary, or familial, or may occur without such a relationship and are called *sporadic.* A sporadic disease may be the result of a change in various genes and would then be called a *mutation.*

Mutations may occur randomly and they may also have a greater likelihood of occurring after exposure to various factors, such as certain drugs, certain chemicals, and certain types of radiation. Some mutations appear to provide some sort of benefit and others can be lethal.

The particular genes that an individual has are called the *genotype.* Every gene does not manifest itself. If the particular product or component that a given gene controls actually develops and is noticed the gene is said to be *expressed.* The total of those genes expressed is called the *phenotype.* A phenotype is made up of a number of *traits,* such as eye color. Certain environmental factors may be needed for a particular gene to be expressed, as mentioned earlier.

A person's genotype has contributions from the father and mother in equal parts. Genes are contained on *chromosomes* and a normal human individual has 46 chromosomes that are really 23 pairs. Each parent provides a set of 23 chromosomes.

If each parent contributes a gene that designates a different manifestation of the same trait, usually only one of these genes will be expressed, since generally one manifestation is dominant and the other is recessive.

Eye color transmission is a good example of these concepts. To understand eye color transmission one needs to know that brown is dominant over blue. Thus, the only way a person can have blue eyes is if she inherits the gene for blue eyes from each parent, since blue is recessive. If the person had inherited one gene for blue eyes and one gene for brown eyes or both genes were for brown eyes, he would have brown eyes.

In order for a parent to transmit a gene for blue eyes, he or she must have at least one gene for blue eyes. The parent may actually have brown eyes, even if one gene is for blue eyes, since the other gene could be for brown eyes. Since brown is the dominant gene, brown would be the color expressed.

It is possible to predict the chances of a child having a certain eye color if one knows which genes the parents have. If both parents have only genes for brown eyes, all the children will have brown eyes. If both parents have only genes for blue eyes, all the children will have blue eyes. If each parent has one gene of each type, the child has a 75 percent chance of having brown eyes. Even though 75 percent of the children will have brown eyes, only 25 percent of all the children will have both genes be for brown eyes. Fifty percent of the children will have brown eyes and yet have one of their two eye-color genes be for blue eyes. They are called *carriers* for the blue trait.

A diagram helps to clarify the possibilities. The two genes that one parent has are listed at the top and those of the other parent are at the side. The various combinations that a child from these parents might have are listed in the boxes. Other combinations can be tried.

Parent's Genes	**Brown**	**Blue**
Brown	Brown Brown	Blue Brown
Blue	Brown Blue	Blue Blue

It can be understood now why a child may have blue eyes even if both parents have brown eyes. Both parents would have had to have been carriers for the blue trait.

There are two chromosomes, designated X and Y, that determine sexual differences, among other traits. A female has two X chromosomes and a male has one X and one Y chromosome. For genes on these chromosomes, called *sex-linked,* the situation is slightly different, since a male can have a recessive trait expressed only when it is on one X chromosome (since he has only one), whereas a female would need to have the recessive trait on both X chromosomes for it to be expressed.

Certain types of color blindness are good examples of this. The most common type of color blindness is caused by a gene on the X chromosome. This is the reason that color blindness is seen more frequently in males. It is possible for a female to be color blind, however, if both X chromosomes have the gene for color blindness. Such an event could happen in 50 percent of female children if the female parent was a carrier and the male parent was color blind. (Color vision is discussed in Chapter 2.)

Some traits, whether they are dominant or recessive, are called normal variants since it does not seem to make too much difference which trait is expressed. Eye color is an example. Other traits are called abnormal because when they are present and expressed, a disease of one sort or another is seen. Inherited diseases may be dominant, recessive, or sex-linked. The inheritance of these diseases is the same as discussed before for the inheritance of traits in these categories.

Non-sex-linked recessive diseases can be disturbing since neither parent may have expressed the disease, yet both may be carriers. There may not have been any prior known cases in the family, since people could have been carriers for several generations without the disease being expressed. In this case, 25 percent of the children will have the disease expressed. Consanguinity, that is, mating between close relatives, increases the incidence of expression of such recessive traits because there is a greater chance of both parents being carriers.

In dominant and sex-linked diseases it is generally possible to find a family history of the disease. However, knowledge of the presence or absence of the trait or disease is needed for three or more generations to establish a hereditary tendency. It should be noted that sex-linked diseases may commonly skip generations since a male with the trait on his X chromosome will pass the trait to his daughters but not to his sons. Neither his sons nor his daughters will have the trait, assuming his mate does not have the trait. However, his daughters will be carriers and may pass the trait to their sons, who would then have the trait or disease that their grandfather had.

The actual situation is really much more complex. Whether a trait is expressed depends not only on how normal the particular component is but also how much of that component is produced. Thus, the recessive gene may produce a normal product but just not enough of it, so that the total amount produced by both corresponding recessive genes is insufficient. This can account for various degrees of severity of inherited diseases from person to person. In the case of eye color, the recessive trait, which is expressed as a blue eye color, is really just caused by a decreased amount of the normal pigment.

There are many examples of each type of inherited disease. As a general rule, the incidence of these inherited diseases is comparatively low. If you have such a disease, your ophthalmologist can provide genetic counseling so that you will have some idea of the chances of passing the disease to your children. He or she can also give you the prognosis. Examples of dominant diseases affecting the eye include dominant drusen and Wagner's hyaloid retinal degeneration. Examples of recessive diseases include gyrate atrophy and Leber's congenital amaurosis. Examples of sex-linked diseases include X-linked retinoschisis and choroideremia. Many other examples could be given.

Some diseases are transmitted in a variety of ways. Retinitis pigmentosa is an example. It may be transmitted as a dominant, recessive, or sex-linked disease. These different types have different degrees of severity, and even within one type the degree of severity varies. Retinitis pigmentosa is a disease of certain cells that provide nourishment for the retina. Early symptoms include problems with night vision and peripheral vision. A test called an electroretinogram can help differentiate these types at an early stage of development. This is useful for prognostic and genetic counseling purposes. Currently, considerable research is being done with regard to this disease. The National Retinitis Pigmentosa Foundation is a good source of information:

National Retinitis Pigmentosa Foundation
8331 Mindale Circle
Baltimore, Maryland 21207
Telephone: (301) 655-1011

Other diseases have what is termed *multifactorial inheritance*. This means that the inheritance patterns are not as precise as previously discussed, since many different genes are involved. Examples of diseases in this category would include glaucoma, strabismus, and refractive errors. This is why these problems are said to have a tendency to be inherited rather than a definite inheritance pattern.

Sometimes large sections of a chromosome may be incomplete, duplicated, or malpositioned. These occurrences are generally sporadic and frequently are not compatible with life. One of the more common problems that is compatible with life is Down's syndrome. This problem occurs when there is an extra chromosome number 21, known as trisomy-21. A number of problems are noted with this disease with the body in general, such as decreased mental development, and the eye in particular, such as strabismus. Some children with this problem are affected to a greater extent than others.

An example of a disease that is sometimes associated with a malpositioned part of a chromosome is a tumor of the retina seen in childhood called retinoblastoma. Most cases of retinoblastoma are not inherited, but in cases where it is, your ophthalmologist can provide genetic counseling as to the chances of other children developing the disease.

Sometimes chromosomal abnormalities and other inherited problems can be detected in the fetal stage of development by a technique called amniocentesis. This technique involves the withdrawal of a small amount of fluid from the amniotic sac, which is the sac surrounding the fetus. Cells from the fetus that are not needed and that are floating in the fluid can be analyzed to see if a problem may be present. This procedure is usually performed only if there is a higher risk of a certain abnormality, because the procedure does have some risk. If certain abnormalities are present, termination of the pregnancy is advised.

A number of other problems are classified as developmental abnormalities. The causes of these problems are not known. Examples of this type include a coloboma and persistent hyperplastic primary vitreous.

Your ophthalmologist is a good source of further information about any of these disorders or types of problems. He or she can tell you about various treatments and prognoses, if known. Another source for this type of information is listed below:

National Foundation—March of Dimes
Genetic Counseling Services
1275 Mamaroneck Avenue
White Plains, New York 10605
Telephone: (419) 428-7100

CHAPTER 7

Undergoing Eye Surgery

Eye surgery has become much safer in the past 10 to 20 years. Some of the reasons for this include the use of the operating microscope; the use of much thinner and less allergy-producing suture material; the use of sharper and smaller needles; the use of smaller, more delicate instruments; and administration of various drugs to produce more rapid changes in certain instances. Many procedures are now performed under local anesthesia only. In local anesthesia only the immediate area to be operated on is anesthetized. Medications may be given to make you drowsy but you will not be completely asleep, as in general anesthesia.

Most eye surgery is what is called elective, that is, it is scheduled in advance since it is not an emergency. Thus, there is time to seek another opinion before the surgery is scheduled. If you would like to have another opinion you should not hesitate to obtain one. You may wish to seek such an opinion by yourself or to ask your ophthalmologist to recommend another person for this purpose.

You will be told when and where to report. Generally this is the admissions desk at the particular hospital. You may prefer a private room, which is somewhat more expensive. On the other hand, particularly if both eyes are patched, you may prefer a semiprivate room so that you may have someone with whom to talk. In many hospitals, an effort is made to have all patients undergoing eye surgery located on the same floor, so your roommate may have a similar problem.

Many eye operations are performed on an outpatient basis. This means that you go to the hospital in the morning, have the surgery, and go home in the afternoon. If you are having surgery as an outpatient, you will not have a regular hospital room. Instead, you will be allowed to go home directly from the recovery area. Your doctor will decide if this is appropriate for your problem. Specific instructions will be given to you if outpatient surgery is recommended.

Preparing children mentally and emotionally in advance for surgery is an important part of the procedure. Surgery on children is often performed on an outpatient basis. Children should have the process explained to them to the extent that they are able to understand it. They should be told that the eye is not removed from the head, for example, and that they should be able to see after the operation. They should be encouraged to discuss any fears they may have. Various positive aspects of the experience can be emphasized. For example, they may be told that there will be other children there, that they can talk into the anesthesia machine, and that they will get their favorite ice cream after surgery. They should understand that the surgery is not punishment for misbehavior. Your ophthalmologist can give you more information on how to handle this.

You will want to wash your hair and face carefully beginning several days before surgery, or as your ophthalmologist recommends. An eyelid infection, for example, may make it preferable to postpone elective surgery. You need to bring only personal effects, such as toilet articles. When you check in at the hospital various forms must be filled out. If you have health insurance, the appropriate names and numbers should be readily available. If you do not have any insurance, you should discuss this with your ophthalmologist before the surgery is scheduled so that you will not be liable for an expensive hospitalization bill that was not anticipated. Alternative arrangements may be available.

Depending on your age, medical problems, and type of procedure to be done, various tests may be performed when you check in, including such things as a chest x-ray, an electrocardiogram, and blood tests. In some places, these tests and other tests specifically for the eye are done a few days before the scheduled admission date.

You will be taken to your room and a nurse will ask you general questions and show you various facilities and explain how to summon help.

Sometime before surgery you will be asked to sign a consent to the operation, which basically gives your doctor permission to perform the surgery. Among other things, it states that you are aware of various risks, alternative courses of treatment, and possibilities of success. These items should have been discussed with your doctor before surgery was scheduled and should not come as a surprise. However, if you do have questions or doubts, be sure to ask. Many of these sorts of risks and alternatives have been discussed in the preceding chapters of this book.

Before surgery your doctor will arrange for an assistant surgeon, if the procedure requires one. You may not meet the assistant until you see him or her in the operating room. An anesthesiologist may be needed and arrangements for one to present will also have been made. If an anesthesiologist is needed you will meet him or her before the operation, usually the day before; he or she will discuss the anesthesia procedure and also have you sign a consent for anesthesia. You should ask any questions or make any requests that you may have. Your doctor will check the results of any laboratory tests and write various orders and notes in your chart.

There are several things you can do to help make the operation be even smoother and safer. The most important thing to do is to *relax.* If you need help going to sleep the night before, don't be afraid to ask for medication. If you have any questions, be sure to ask them.

The night before surgery, drops may be placed in your eye and your eyelashes may be trimmed. The lashes grow back in a few weeks and it is sometimes best to keep them out of the way to prevent them from contaminating the area being operated on.

On the day of surgery you may be given an injection to help you relax and for some procedures you may be given a syrupy liquid to drink. It is important that you *not* eat or drink anything after midnight before surgery, even if it is on an outpatient basis, unless it is a medication specifically given to you to take or you are instructed otherwise. If the surgery is scheduled for late in the day, you may be allowed to have some liquids in the morning. The reasons you are not allowed to eat is that you may vomit the food and inhale it, thus causing you to choke. Just before you go to the operating room you should move your bowels and empty your bladder if you need to do so.

In the operating room you will be positioned on a table. If you are not comfortable, say so and an effort will be made to try to solve the problem. Various monitors will be attached and an intravenous (IV) line started, in case any medication needs to be given. If the operation is under local anesthesia, the anesthetic will be injected around your eye. Several injection sites may be used. These injections are *not* placed into the eye. After an initial sting, you should not feel anything. If you have pain, say so. If general anesthesia is used, you will be completely asleep. During the operation, the eye having the surgery does *not* see what is happening because of the anesthetic. The anesthetic affects all types of nerves including the ones that transmit pain, the ones that transmit vision, and also the ones that go to the muscles that move your eye. You will be covered with sterile drapes after your eye is thoroughly washed and an oxygen line will be placed near your nose so you can breathe easily. It is important that you lie still after the drapes are placed so that you don't contaminate anything.

Operating times vary, but most eye operations take from one to three hours. If the operation is done under local anesthesia, you may be given instructions from time to time, such as not to move. The eyeball is *not* removed from the head and later placed back in position. The only time the eyeball is removed is if that is the surgery that is to be performed. In that case it is not placed back.

At the end of the operation a patch and shield will, depending on the operation, usually be applied to your eye and you will be placed on a cart to take you to the recovery room and then back to your room. In some instances both eyes may be covered even if only one eye was operated on.

For the first day after surgery you should rest quietly. Depending on the operation you may be able to go to the bathroom with help. You can usually eat if you feel like it and medications for pain, sleep, and your bowels will be ordered; however, generally you must ask for them by pushing the button to call the nurse, if you need them.

You will have a gradual increase in activity until you are discharged. Then you will be given instructions on how to take care of your eye and when to come to your ophthalmologist's office for followup. Many times, most, if not all, of the sutures are of the absorbable type and do not need to be removed. Those that do need to be removed can frequently be easily removed in your ophthalmologist's office with only a drop of topical anesthetic. Children frequently have all absorbable sutures, depending on the surgical procedure.

You should take care not to lift or carry any items that weigh more than one pound and should be extra careful not to contaminate your eye when bathing. Bend down by bending your knees and not your waist. Try to avoid being constipated by taking a laxative, if needed. Try not to rub the operated eye or to sleep on the operated eye. It may be necessary to wear a shield or glasses, depending on the operation. Do *not* engage in vigorous exercise or go swimming until given permission to do so. Most people need to be rather careful for the first month after surgery and are usually not considered to be fully rehabilitated before three months or more have gone by.

Any questions should be written down so you won't forget them. Do not be afraid to ask your doctor any question.

CHAPTER 8

New Procedures and Techniques of Eye Care

A number of new procedures and techniques are currently being investigated in ophthalmology. Some of them have already been discussed in some detail. It is important to remember that a new procedure is not necessarily a better one. On the other hand, each procedure commonly used today was at one time a new procedure. The criteria for deciding which procedures will ultimately become routine are based on the scientific method. Until proper controlled trials of the new procedure comparing it with the old one have been done, it is not possible to say if it is a better way or if in fact it is actually a worse way and perhaps more harmful and more expensive. Since many of the problems that can develop with new techniques do not become apparent for years and sometimes decades, the problem of long-term results is a real one. Thus, acceptance of new procedures to the point that they become routine is a slow process.

Frequently, animals are used to test various new ideas regarding treatments. Unfortunately, an animal model is not a perfect model for the situation in human beings. A new drug that appears to solve a particular problem quite well in an animal may have an unforeseen or unmeasurable side effect. For example, it is hard to measure the side effect of mental depression in a rabbit for an otherwise quite acceptable drug. In addition, a rabbit's eye is not exactly like a human eye. To name only two examples, the lens is proportionately larger than the human lens and certain cells in the cornea (the endothelial cells) can regenerate in a rabbit but not in a human. On the other hand, a rabbit is a good model for testing absorption of drugs when given as a drop or periocular injection. Other animal models have different advantages and disadvantages. Sometimes there is no animal model that is even partially acceptable, for example, in certain rare, inherited human disorders. This obviously makes it more difficult to tell if a proposed treatment is helpful or perhaps harmful.

Once animal research has shown a technique or drug to appear promising, it is tested on human volunteers. These studies on humans are called clinical trials and are set up using the principles of the scientific method. Additional factors, such as ethical aspects, must also be considered.

Those patients who are participating in the trial need to know that fact and need to be informed of the known risks and alternatives. They must sign an informed consent document. The investigators running the trial need to arrange what is called a randomized controlled clinical trial.

This is sometimes called a double-blind study. This means that the patients are assigned randomly to either the control group or the experimental group. The patients and the doctors do not get a choice as to which group a patient is assigned. There are various techniques for ensuring this. The double-blind part does not refer to the patient's vision. It refers to the fact that the patients must not know which group they are in and the people who test the effect on the patients must not know who is in which group. Various codes can be used to allow the patients to be identified without violating the double-blind principle.

A simple example can clarify this. If a drug, given as an eye drop, is being tested to see if it lowers the pressure inside the eye, the experimental group would be given the drug that is being tested and the control group would be given what is termed a placebo, which in this case could be a drop of water. The placebo has previously been determined not to affect the problem under investigation. The patients do not know if they received the drug or the placebo. The people who subsequently measure the pressure, according to the protocol, also do not know which patient received the drug and which received the placebo. The people who analyze the results do, however, know. Codes are used to provide confidentiality.

In a clinical trial an effort is made to try to match the two groups in order to eliminate other variables as much as possible. Age, sex, previous history, other medical problems, and so forth are factors that might be considered. It is obviously not possible to run a clinical trial according to the strict criteria used for nonhuman research. However, the better matched the two groups are and the more perfectly the principles of the scientific method are observed, the more reliable the results will be.

In some cases it is necessary to expend considerable effort to test various hypotheses. These clinical trials are run on a nationwide basis with very precise protocols. One recent such clinical trial, directed by the National Eye Institute, was devised to test the effectiveness of laser treatment for certain problems associated with diabetes mellitus. A subsequent study is currently underway to test other variables and techniques along the same lines, for example, using the laser to treat these problems earlier. These studies involve the cooperation of hundreds of people and considerable attention is given to having adequate controls and uniformly followed protocols. Studies like these are randomized controlled clinical trials. Information about these studies and many others that are currently underway can be obtained from the National Eye Institute:

National Eye Institute, Information Office
National Institutes of Health
Building 31, Room 6A25
Bethesda, Maryland 20205
Telephone: (301) 496-5248

NEW METHODS OF CORRECTING A REFRACTIVE ERROR

Many of the new techniques relate to trying to find a better way to correct refractive errors. The usual method is the use of common eyeglasses, as discussed earlier. However, for large refractive errors, such as after a cataract extraction, glasses give distortions that one would like to minimize. There are newer ways of grinding such higher power lenses to minimize some of these distortions. Such lenses are termed aspherical. The term comes from the fact that the lens is not spherical. The changes from the symmetry of the sphere are an attempt to neutralize some of these distortions. Various trade names are used for such lenses, and there are some differences in the way they are made aspherical.

Contact lenses (hard, soft, and continuous wear) and intraocular lenses have been used in the last several years as alternatives and were discussed previously in Chapters 2 and 4.

Glasses with a bifocal correction that do not have a "line" visible, continuous curve lenses, were also discussed in Chapter 2.

Recently, some people have tried to surgically correct a refractive error by changing the power of the cornea itself, a technique called *refractive keratoplasty*. One method is to first remove part of the cornea. The corneal section is then frozen and a lathe is used to shave the cornea in such a way as to change the curve and hence the power. The corneal section is then defrosted and sewn back into position. This procedure is called *keratomileusis*. Sometimes an extra section of tissue is inserted into the center of the cornea to change the power and this procedure is called *keratophakia*. These procedures are not simple; they require complex equipment and carry significant potential risk. How real these risks will in fact turn out to be is not yet known.

An even more recent technique is called *radial keratotomy* and involves making small but fairly deep cuts on the cornea. The shape and thus the power of the cornea will change, but as yet not in an absolutely predictable manner. Other problems noted with radial keratotomy include such things as significant glare, rapid reversion to the original refractive error, problems in subsequently wearing contact lenses to correct residual refractive errors, recurrent corneal abrasions, corneal scars, fluctuating visual acuity throughout the day, and vision worse than prior to surgery. Various combinations of these problems have been noted in some patients who have had this procedure. Other potential risks include perforation of the eye, with risk of an infection inside the eye that can often lead to total loss of vision.

These techniques are generally thought to be experimental and the long-term consequences of each are not known. In addition, the technique and instrumentation is changing fairly rapidly. These procedures are done in only a relatively small number of places.

Other surgical advances are being made in the treatment of cataracts and glaucoma. These have been discussed in Chapter 4.

NEW DRUGS

Many new drugs have recently been introduced. For example, drugs that are more effective in treating herpes simplex virus infections of the cornea are now available and drugs with fewer side effects are available for the treatment of glaucoma. A new type of drug delivery system was discussed in Chapter 4. The newer drugs tend to be more expensive and if the older ones are working satisfactorily your ophthalmologist may choose not to change your medication.

A number of other drugs, procedures, and techniques are still being tried and developed in laboratories. Hopefully, many of these will prove to be useful and safe for treatment of various disorders of the eye. Your ophthalmologist becomes aware of these developments and the results of various experiments by reading scientific journals, attending meetings, taking courses, and discussing these developments and other problems with his fellow ophthalmologists, physicians, and scientists. Continuing education is a very real part of an ophthalmologist's life. Many states even require evidence of a certain amount of such education after the formal training period is over, in order to renew the license to practice medicine. If you have any questions about current research, do not hesitate to ask your ophthalmologist.

CHAPTER 9

Eye Care Checklist

This last chapter basically provides a summary of important points to remember in the care of your eyes. All of them were discussed in previous chapters.

1. Know the emergency procedures discussed in the first chapter. Remember that for liquids, powders, or chemicals that accidentally get into the eye, much water should be used to rinse the eye as quickly as possible. Substances like metal fragments that may have penetrated the globe should not be rinsed. See an ophthalmologist after any such injury to the eye or eyelids to treat this injury and ensure that no other damage has occurred.
2. Use proper protection for your eyes. This might include goggles, shields, or sunglasses, depending on the situation. Don't be lazy and forget to use your protective gear.
3. Keep dangerous items away from children. You must "child-proof" your home. This includes locking up potentially harmful chemicals, such as cleaning solutions and powders. In addition, sharp objects such as scissors and knives must be put

in safe places where children can't get to them. Toys should be bought with concern for their potential danger to the eyes.

4. Only put medications in your eye that are specifically designed to be used for the eye. Do not use old or contaminated medicines.
5. Know what drugs and medications and the amounts of each that you take not just for your eyes but for any purpose. It is convenient to keep a list with this information that can be shown to any doctor you may visit.
6. Know what, if any, drugs you are allergic to and what happened to you when you took the drug. Be sure that you let every doctor you visit know about these reactions.
7. Keep a copy of your eyeglass or contact lens prescription and specifications, if you wear them, in a safe place, and another copy with your documents if you take a trip. It may be advisable to have a spare pair of glasses or contact lenses, depending on your prescription and where you are traveling.
8. Keep your glasses clean and in adjustment. Follow your doctor's advice to keep your contact lenses clean.
9. Take medicines that are prescribed in the way in which they were prescribed. In other words, follow the directions.
10. Keep an adequate supply of prescribed medicines so that you don't run out.
11. Eat properly and get sufficient sleep and exercise.
12. Keep your eyelids, face, hair, and scalp clean.
13. Avoid things that are known to cause problems for you, such as certain makeup preparations or powders, even if other people do not have problems with these items.
14. Keep other diseases you may have in as good control as possible, such as high blood pressure and diabetes mellitus.
15. If you have a problem that may be inherited, have other family members also see an ophthalmologist to be checked.
16. Tell other doctors you visit about any problems with your eyes that you are being treated for, such as glaucoma.
17. Be wary of magical and unproven cures. Do not delay diagnosis and treatment of potentially serious disorders because of them. Keep the principles of the scientific method in mind when you evaluate such ideas.

18. If you notice any enlarging mass on your eyelids, you should see an ophthalmologist immediately.
19. If you have sudden pain, haloes, discharge, loss of vision, loss of visual field, or other suspicious change of vision you should call an ophthalmologist.
20. If you need surgery, approach the prospect optimistically. Keep in mind the recent advances that have led to an increased rate of successful surgery.
21. Keep all your appointments for follow-up examinations.
22. Have a regular, complete medical eye examination by an ophthalmologist. Be aware of the differences between an ophthalmologist and other eye care providers. Realize that an ophthalmologist can also prescribe eyeglasses and contact lenses, in addition to diagnosing and treating medical and surgical eye problems.
23. Keep a list of any questions you may have and do not *ever* be afraid to ask them, no matter how simple, silly, or stupid you may think they might be. Your ophthalmologist should be able to answer most questions you may have about new developments or other problems. If this information is not sufficient, he or she can refer you to another source or person who may be able to help. The American Academy of Ophthalmology and the National Eye Institute are good additional sources of information. They publish a number of items regarding care and treatment of the eyes that may be helpful. Their addresses are listed below:

Public and Professional Education Committee
American Academy of Ophthalmology
P.O. Box 7424
San Francisco, California 94120

National Eye Institute, Information Office
National Institutes of Health
Building 31, Room 6A25
Bethesda, Maryland 20205
Telephone: (301) 496-5248

Index